The Family Health History Workbook

The Family Health History Workbook

Marnie Mahoney
Ronnie Lichtman, CNM

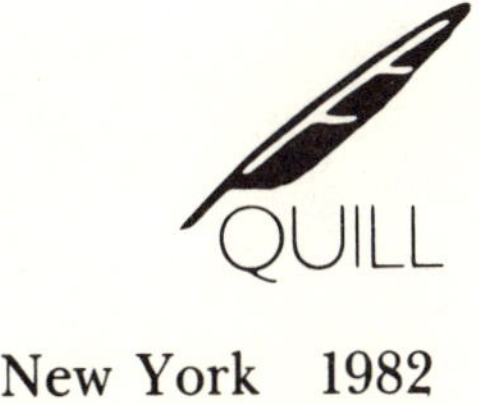

QUILL

New York   1982

Library of Congress Cataloging in Publication Data

Mahoney, Martha
    The family health history workbook.

    Includes index.
    1. Medical records—Forms.   2. Family—Health and
hygiene—Forms.   I. Lichtman, Ronnie.   II. Title.
[R864.M33   1982]   613   82-7679
ISBN 0-688-01005-9 (pbk.)   AACR2

Text design: Levavi & Levavi

Printed in the United States of America

First Quill Edition

1 2 3 4 5 6 7 8 9 10

We dedicate this book to the parents and the
children of the world, especially to our parents

Jeanne Adleman-Mahoney   Gertrude Lichtman
William B. Mahoney   Emanuel Lichtman

who gave us not only love, but their vision
of a better world and their steadfast example
in its pursuit,

and to our children, in trust and hope,

Amanda Leah Crockett and Jeffrey Liam Crockett,
who inspired this work, and to future children,
who will bring new inspirations

Acknowledgments

There are two people without whom this book would not have been—Eileen Lottman and Jeanne Adleman-Mahoney. Their belief in this project made it possible. They have our endless gratitude.

The following individuals offered ideas and suggestions, provided information and/or comments on the manuscript. Their help has made a better book: Amy S. Abrams, Nikki Alexander, M.S.W., Suzanne Arms, Velma Campbell, M.D., Suzanne Danilson, Vickie Gordon, Joseph Halbach, M.D., Gertrude and Emanuel Lichtman, Steven Lichtman, Joan Mahoney, William Mahoney, Shifra B. Miller, Donna Myhre, Judith Pasternak, Kent Treadway, M.D., Dorothy Zellner, and Suellen Zima.

We'd like to thank the authors whose material we have adapted or reprinted in various sections of the book. Their names are mentioned where their work appears.

A special thank-you goes to the people from whom we've learned throughout the years. First, there were the many women in the women's health movement. There have been teachers, colleagues, and students. In particular, Ronnie has warm appreciation for the faculty and students of the Columbia University midwifery program and the original staff of the North Central Bronx Hospital midwifery service. Our greatest learning has come in the course of our work—for Ronnie, from those families whose pregnancies and births she was privileged to share, and for Marnie, from the courage and experience of her friends and coworkers in the garment factories of New Orleans.

These acknowledgments must include friends and family members who have given us the love and support so needed to write. To list each person in both our lives would take far too long, and some have been mentioned above. There are a few whose names cannot be excluded, however. They are Laura Brenner, Vernet Brown, Liz Slechta Christopher, Debby D'Amico-Samuels, Denise Ford, Maxine Jones, Allan Lichtman, Donald Mahoney, Sydelle Postman, Georgette Schneer, Sandra Stimpson, Viv Sutherland, and, with special love, Amanda and Jeffrey Crockett.

Finally, we wish to thank Robert Bender and Howard Cady, the two editors with whom we've had the good fortune to work.

All errors, omissions, and opinions are, of course, our own.

Contents

5. *CHILDHOOD*   **251**

LIST OF RECORD-KEEPING CHARTS

LIST OF SAMPLE CHARTS

Introduction

This is a book you will write. Part of it has already been written, in your family's history and in your life choices. Other parts you will create—as routinely as writing a shopping list, and as creatively as bearing and rearing children.

The Family Health History Workbook is designed for you to explore and record the many and diverse elements that affect the health of your family. This will lead through the obvious—surgeries, family illness, childhood immunizations, and allergies. And it will lead further—for example, on-the-job chemical exposure, nutrition, exercise, and stress.

The idea for a *Family Health History Workbook* grew out of the increased popular interest and participation in health care that has developed over the last fifteen years. We health consumers have discovered, often to our dismay, that doctors' records aren't the complete, precise resources we had imagined. Our life-styles have changed. We move more frequently, often over great distances, so access to records of past care has become more difficult. And increased specialization means that often each family member is seeing several different practitioners at once, so a family's care-givers can include an obstetrician, a dentist, an orthopedist, a pediatrician, and an optometrist. Clinic patients may see several different practitioners within each specialty.

Even our vocabulary has changed. Technologically, it has come to include such terms as CAT scan, ultrasound, and chemotherapy. Our everyday vocabulary has changed as well. We now speak of "wellness" instead of illness and discuss "holistic health." Even the old GP (general practitioner) has become a specialist in family practice.

Many of these changes are the result of a conscious and growing health movement which has its roots in the civil rights and women's struggles. This movement has two distinct trends—self-help and the demand for social change. This record-keeping book reflects thinking from both trends. It will help us take advantage of developing technology without letting this technology depersonalize us.

Your *Family Health History Workbook* is to be read and used for many years. It is divided into sections which reflect health needs at different life stages. The importance of each section will change with time. We suggest you survey the book's contents and carefully read the section "How to Use This Book" (p. 21).

SELF-HELP VS. CHANGING THE SYSTEM

Self-help can be looked at in many ways. Its broadest meaning refers to the public's increased knowledge and understanding of health issues. At the other end of the self-help continuum are self-taught women's groups which practice gynecological self-examination and do research. The recent popular interest in jogging can be seen as part of the self-help trend, as can the huge leap forward in nutritional consciousness.

The main emphasis of self-help is on the responsibility and participation of the individual. One of its greatest strengths is the return of decision-making from the health professional to the consumer. This process has also worked for groups. For example, women's self-help organizations have defined and carried out their own research on menstrual extractions.

Self-help recognizes that the individual's own action—or inaction—can have a profound effect on health. This leads to a great emphasis on wellness and can contribute to prevention of some serious disorders. Early detection is also a benefit, as in breast self-examination. Finally, self-help promotes a positive self-image; it removes the body from the realm of fear and mystery.

Obviously, keeping your family health-history records can be seen as part of the self-help trend. It serves as a communication tool, gathering information from your family and your own records to give to your practitioner and to increase your own awareness. It helps organize the information you need to obtain from your practitioner as well. For your future needs and those of your children, it can provide information to let you "backtrack" when new medical knowledge emerges, checking against the treatments and medications you have received in the past.

Some self-help supporters claim that it contributes to improvement in accepted medical practice. We question whether it is actually the self-help process that brings about change, or whether progress comes from direct advocacy programs.

Since the late sixties many activists, local organizations, and national lobbying groups have come forward to demand more responsive health care. They have had—and continue to have—many criticisms of the existing health-care delivery system. One of the most widespread and serious of these criticisms is the inequality of services. This inequality is being sharpened by government policies that demonstrate an increasing unwillingness to meet people's basic needs.

Poor people and members of minority groups have been frequent victims of "care" in public-health clinics and municipal hospitals where they have been used without their consent for medical research and to teach medical students. Government hospitals are essentially staffed by rotating groups of doctors-in-training. The more experienced physicians are teaching—supervising—and are not often seen by the patients.

Women have been treated patronizingly by male health professionals and have often undergone unnecessary surgery and dehumanizing treatment. Poor or minority-group women have been subject to entirely different diagnoses when they have presented the same symptoms as middle-class or rich white women. Pelvic inflammatory disease, for example, has been a "lower-class" diagnosis because it can develop from venereal disease; endometriosis has been the diagnosis given to the elite with the same symptoms. Other diseases, such as sickle-cell anemia, have been virtually ignored for many years because they affect mainly blacks, and they still receive inadequate support for research.

If we consider that we live not just in the United States but in the world, we see more and greater inequities. Poor people in the Third World have been subjected to imposed medical experimentation. Unknowing Latin American women, for example, were used to test the effectiveness and safety of birth-control pills.

The underdeveloped world is used by American companies as a virtual "dumping ground" for drugs and other hazardous substances, some not approved by the U.S. Food and Drug Administration. A recent example is the distribution of Depo-Provera ("the shot") for birth control. Depo-Provera provides long-term protection against pregnancy. However, it is believed to have too many potentially life-threatening side effects to win approval for use as a birth-control method in this country.

In the past twenty years, giant multinational corporations have created a worldwide, billion-dollar, never-ending market for infant formula. The consequences in terms of infant health have been dramatic and tragic. Serious infections occur in the many areas where necessary facilities for sterilization of formula are nonexistent. Malnutrition is common where families cannot afford to purchase enough formula to supply adequate calories and nutrients. Infection and malnutrition all too often lead to death. The infant-formula issue has provoked a boycott movement and international protests.

Inside the United States, as the movement for change in the health-care system developed, people searched for explanations of the inequities confronting them. First, many questioned whether health should be a profit-making industry. Obvious contradictions between public need and private profit existed, as evidenced by the reluctance of drug companies to produce and market drugs with low profit margins. Another example is the growing expense of health care stimulated by increasing reliance on expensive but profitable technology.

Even among those who accept health care as a business, questions have been raised as to whether fees should be paid for individual services. In clinics, the effect of a fee-for-service system is that practitioners must often weigh the benefits of tests and treatments against their cost, either to the patient or to the government. In private practice, it has the opposite effect: practitioners may perform unnecessary tests, such as X rays, to pay for the equipment needed for indicated tests. Unscrupulous practitioners even order unnecessary treatments, such as surgeries, to collect fees. These acute injustices gave rise to demands for change on many fronts.

Civil Rights and Health

One of the most fundamental battlegrounds has always been the area of civil rights. Abortion or pro-choice issues, the prevention of sterilization abuse, the needs of the elderly, dignity for gays, and mobility for the disabled have all become areas for organizing for change. Perhaps the most profound transformation has occurred in the public's consciousness of these rights. Specific advances have included legalization of abortion and some protective regulations on sterilization. Setbacks have also occurred, such as loss of federal funding for Medicaid abortions.

Municipal Hospitals and Clinics

During this same period, municipal hospitals have become the focus of community activism in many forms. Protection, expansion, and improvement of services have been the goals of communities dependent on these institutions. At times, hospital workers have joined with neighborhood groups in pursuit of better conditions for employees and patients alike. Here, too, concessions have been made. Patient-advocacy programs have been implemented in some hospitals. In some areas—New York City, for example—community boards have taken a greater role in planning and decision-making. Some clinics have reorganized so that each patient is seen by the same practitioner at each visit and cared for by that practitioner if hospitalized. We believe this issue, however, will continue to be critical as long as there is one standard of care offered in municipal hospitals and another in private hospitals.

Economic Accessibility of Care

The difference between private and public health care has helped motivate the call for developing payment methods that do not discriminate on the basis of income or wealth. One response to this has been the development of many health maintenance organizations (HMOs). Although they operate for profit, these agencies have at least eliminated fees for service. Instead, a yearly payment entitles members to most needed care, including preventive examinations.

On the legislative front, proposals have been introduced in Congress for the creation of National Health Insurance, and there has even been a bill proposing the creation of a National Health Service. National Health Insurance would pay for services that are now paid for by individuals, private health-insurance companies, or existing state and national programs. It would not change the basic fee-for-service system or eliminate health care for profit. Under a National Health Service, fees would not be paid for care. Rather, all health workers would be employed by the service and receive a salary, as teachers do in our system of free public education.

Occupational Health

In recent years the movement for health protection in the workplace has spread and grown to almost every major industry and even some white-collar and professional jobs. Inside the mines and the textile mills, movements developed for better prevention and treatment for lung disease. Scandals exposed factory owners who concealed hazardous chemical exposures from their workers. Often the dangers were discovered only after tragic consequences such as the onset of sterility or cancer. The demand for health and safety protection increased in importance in union negotiations and in some areas, particularly the coal mines, became the focal issue in workers' strikes. The creation of the Occupational Safety and Health Administration (OSHA) was a response to this movement. OSHA has been criticized by labor for having inadequate enforcement provisions and for imposing token fines on companies who can well afford these penalties. However, current trends in government are toward weaker protection and threaten OSHA's very existence.

Abuse-Victim Support Services

For several years, it almost seemed as if new sets of victims were being discovered at every turn. In fact, education and consciousness-raising were removing the stigma of guilt and shame associated with having been beaten, raped, or abused. Institutions to assist abuse victims, such as battered women's shelters and rape crisis lines, have developed alongside self-help measures: support groups and peer counseling. Demands have been made for increased sensitivity from practitioners, especially from police and emergency personnel. Some police departments and hospitals have responded by training special teams to protect victims from further psychological harm and to secure proper evidence so that legal action, including prosecution, can be undertaken.

Education and persistent organizing are beginning to change the public perspective that held the victim responsible. Research has begun, and a body of knowledge on prevention and treatment for abuse victims is emerging.

Iatrogenic (Practitioner-Induced) Disorders

Iatrogenic disorders are those caused directly by health care. This may seem like a contradiction in terms, but it really isn't: Think of a patient who develops a vitamin deficiency on a hospital diet, or a man with borderline high blood pressure whose medication leads to impotence, or a baby born prematurely because of a poorly timed repeat Cesarean section.

Some of the most publicized medical scandals of our time have been iatrogenic disorders. These include the thalidomide babies of the early sixties and more recently the discoveries about the devastating effects of diethylstilbestrol (DES) on the children of the women who took it during pregnancy.

Several aspects of iatrogenic disorders are currently drawing close attention in the health movement. The first is the extent to which the profit motive intensifies the frequency and severity of the problem. Drug companies put medications on the market whose long-term effects are little known—and practitioners, hurried in the time/profit dynamic of private practice, rely on the literature produced by the drug companies for their prescribing information. Another problem is the enthusiasm of practitioners for intervention at the slightest excuse. Part of this grows out of the nature of medical training, which is aggressively oriented toward treatment with drugs or surgery. It is reinforced by infatuation with new technology, which can lead to the widespread adoption of a new technique such as breast mammography before it is thoroughly tested.

Another significant question for health consumers is that of decision-making. How much information does the patient need to be able to give informed consent to a medical treatment or procedure? (See section on "Informed Consent," p. 116.) And in the end, who has responsibility for making decisions regarding treatment, the practitioner or the consumer?

Considering that some iatrogenic disorders can seriously threaten or alter the patient's life, or necessitate long and costly treatment, the legal problems raised are also important: Whose fault is it? Who pays? If the original treatment fell within accepted medical practice, where does accountability lie? Several class-action suits now pending in the courts seek compensation from drug companies and manufacturers of IUDs who marketed and promoted products with harmful long-range effects. Recent rulings have cleared the way for these cases to be heard in court. But the battle over legal responsibility promises to drag on for many years to come.

Childbirth

A brief look at the history of childbirth practices during the last thirty years illustrates the effectiveness of efforts for change. In 1950, a typical childbirth experience included being isolated from family and friends, alone in a labor bed, probably drugged with amnesiacs and/or narcotics, asleep or barely conscious for birth, and separated from the sleepy newborn. The expectant father, pacing outside the hospital room or drinking with friends nearby, was portrayed as a pathetic or comical figure. The obstetrician was clearly the "star of the show."

Change came about slowly but steadily and was a direct result of the work of families dissatisfied with this kind of care and concerned about its damaging effects on their babies. First came acceptance of education for childbirth. This education has profoundly influenced our beliefs about birth. Women have come to see it as their right to have loving support for labor and delivery and to use medication as they choose, with full awareness of all benefits and side effects. The presence of fathers at birth has become acceptable and indeed desirable. Today, childbirth education is seen as the minimal right of pregnant families.

The increasingly educated public wants control of all aspects of this precious experience. We want warmth and humanity rather than routinized medical treatment of pregnancy and birth, and we want safe and careful use of technology without careless iatrogenesis. (See section on "Labor and Delivery," p. 189.)

Health practitioners and institutions have responded to these demands. Birth centers, in and out of hospitals, have arisen, and an increasing number of midwifery services have been created. These services emphasize noninterference and family rights. New York State has passed an exemplary law requiring that information on benefits and risks of all drugs prescribed during pregnancy, labor, and delivery be given to women. The challenge today is to see that the recognition of rights extends to all families, regardless of income, race, ethnic group, or age.

Holistic Health

The concept of holistic health is one of the new additions to our thinking. It is a philosophy that has generated a variety of self-help groups and has also exerted pressure on accepted medical practices. Advocates of the holistic approach refuse to see a person as a collection of separate symptoms or isolated diseased parts. Practitioners are criticized for thinking of patients as "the kidney stone in Room 5."

Psychological and emotional causes and consequences of disease are given importance equal to the physical. These are, in fact, seen as interrelated. Therapies that consider the body as a total system are most valued. Nutrition, exercise, massage, meditation, and biofeedback have emerged as part of holistic health care.

Organizations dedicated to the holistic approach have sprung up across the nation. Some provide actual services, many function primarily as educational centers, and others act as pressure groups.

The health movement ranges beyond the areas described above. The environmental and antinuclear movements, though having an independent existence, overlap with health issues. The development of hospices, which emphasize dignity, honesty, and the psychological needs of the dying, is another facet of the health movement. Since good health remains important through all stages of life and is affected by many factors, the limits of the health movement are sometimes hard to define.

We hope this book can, in addition to its self-help function, be a tool in the pursuit of quality health care. Despite the popularity and broad attraction of the health movement, when we walk into our practitioner's office we are still individual health consumers. If the needs are present throughout society, they must be met individually. This workbook is designed to help the consumer better evaluate the health care she or he is given. We believe that the better able we are to question and consider health care received, the more responses we are likely to find within the system. Standards of minimum care must be raised to meet the needs of better educated consumers. Less unnecessary care may also result. In fact, through comprehensive family health records, information is made available to practitioners which can increase their awareness of such nontraditional factors as environmental and occupational hazards.

While no one individual is touched by every facet of the health movement, it has affected the lives and thinking of all of us. Our increased involvement in our own wellness and our commitment to participation in any health care we receive are the direct result of increased social consciousness. We hope that the increased self-awareness this book offers can be extended into political and social involvement. We encourage you as individuals to use the information from your own health history, and your experience with the health-care system, to join with others in working toward change in those areas that most affect your life. We firmly believe it is this joint effort and group action that will assure progress toward the recognition of individual rights and the goal of quality health care for all.

How to Use This Book

This is a book to keep and use for many years. Its many sections are designed to represent the needs of various life stages. It is a book that will become part of your family's history. You will refer to it continuously as your children grow; you will take it with you when you move; you will photocopy sections for your children when they leave home.

You can read *The Family Health History Workbook* from cover to cover or you can read it section by section, skipping some to concentrate on the ones that most apply to you. The book is divided into five main parts—Adult Health, Health Issues, Reproductive Health, Childbearing, and Childhood. Within each part, sections are arranged according to topics. Review the Contents and the detailed List of Record-Keeping Charts to familiarize yourself with the many topics covered.

Each section of *The Family Health History Workbook* begins with an introduction which provides you with the information necessary for effective and meaningful record-keeping. Before you begin to fill out any of the charts, carefully read the accompanying introduction. At the end of many sections, such as "Practitioner Visits and Hospitalizations," we have provided additional information to help you with the specifics of filling in the charts. We urge you to read these as well before proceeding with record-keeping.

For almost everybody, the logical place to begin is with the sections "Family History" and "Medical History." In these sections, as in many others, we have provided two charts—one for each adult member of the family. Women can also fill out "Obstetrical History," if applicable. These charts may take the greatest amount of time to complete since they span three generations and cover your entire past life. Once they are filled in, they will be continually referred to, both by you and by your health practitioners.

Other charts, such as "Practitioner Visits and Hospitalizations," will be filled in over a long period of time, although each entry may be quite brief. Some sections, such as "Pregnancy" and "The Postpartum Period," will be used intensely for a relatively short time. The sections "Long-term Illness," "Nutrition," "Exercise," and "Natural Family Planning" give only sample charts since record-keeping in these areas can be a lifetime practice. If you wish to maintain such records, we suggest designing a special notebook to keep as a companion to this book.

Often, more than one chart may be used simultaneously. If you are hospitalized, then you will use the sections "Practitioner Visits and Hospitalizations" and "Informed Consent." In some cases, one section refers you to another since information may overlap. Some sections may seem arbitrarily placed; "Nutrition" is found in Adult Health, for example, even though it includes nutrition in pregnancy, breast-feeding, and childhood, while "Breast-Feeding" is found in the Childhood section since it relates to baby as well as mother. This points up the fact that health care cannot really be separated into parts, but books must be.

At the end of many of the sections, we have listed the names of some books we think are worthwhile. We do not agree with all the information or viewpoints of every reference cited. There are many other excellent books on health care published every day. We encourage further reading on all topics. Scientific knowledge is constantly changing. Controversies abound in all areas. Readers must get further information to formulate their own opinions, judgments, and guidelines for their own health care.

The organization of *The Family Health History Workbook* seems to assume that all families consist of a mother, a father, and two children. Obviously, not all families live this way. Single parenthood is becoming more common. Separation, divorce, death, and remarriage frequently change family patterns. You will revise and expand this book to reflect your own changing family.

The sections "Reproductive History" and "Childbearing" are addressed primarily to women. This was not done because we believe that men should be excluded from these areas. It is merely indicative of the current norm in our society which so often makes reproductive activities the focus of women, since women tend to be the most stable figures in a family. We encourage all men, however, to participate fully in the exciting and crucial tasks of childbearing and child rearing.

As this book evolved, it became clear that much of its emphasis had to be on disease. We firmly believe that illness or its absence is only a fragment of health. Childbirth, for example, is, and should be, a part of life, not of disease. Yet we have included comprehensive charts so you can record any danger signs and complications. Most newborns are healthy, yet we have included a section called "Problems of the Newborn."

This seeming focus on disease came about for a number of reasons. In this age of aggressive medical intervention, not only does disease itself impose possible far-reaching hazards, but so also does its treatment. Even diagnostic tests can be risky. Health practitioners are taught to weigh possible benefits against risks when administering care. However, determinations are often made before risks are fully known or assessed. The decision-making process is rarely shared with the recipient of care. Therefore, we have, on many charts, included extensive information about and large blocks of space for medical tests and treatments. This in no way endorses any of these procedures. The purpose of including examples and details is not to overwhelm but to acquaint you with medical jargon and help you understand medical practices.

Throughout the book, we have tried to balance this heavy medical perspective with space for feelings and with self-help sections such as "Exercise" and "Nutrition." We sincerely hope these sections are regarded as seriously in your record-keeping as are the more medically oriented ones.

Ultimately, the purpose of *The Family Health History Workbook* is not to inspire a morbid or compulsive fascination with your state of health. It is, rather, to increase your awareness and understanding of the workings of your own body. It is to provide you with a basis for evaluation of health problems and health care and, most important, to give you ready reference to valuable information about your family's health.

1.

Adult Health

Family History

Exploring family roots has become an American pastime. Rediscovering family treasures, scouring birth, marriage, and death records to trace genealogies, and taping interviews with living ancestors have all gained recent popularity. Even the most extensive family histories, however, often ignore health history. This is despite the fact that past illnesses may be the most significant part of the history for the family's living members. The purpose of this section is to provide guidelines for recording and evaluating your family's health history.

Gathering the data for a family health history may seem a difficult task to those with large families. It is most important to know about your parents, both sets of grandparents, your own children, sisters and brothers and their children, and aunts and uncles (related by blood, not marriage). Other relatives, such as cousins, can be included if they suffer from a major illness or if their health histories lead you to suspect that something "runs in the family."

We have chosen in the charts that follow to list specific diseases and disorders for which hereditary causes have been demonstrated. Although the science of genetics is continually expanding the knowledge of how a person's health may be affected by genetic factors, the exact role played by inheritance varies and may not always be known or completely understood.

At this time, there are over one thousand diseases or disorders considered to be hereditary and over one thousand others for which hereditary causes are suspected. Geneticists can identify the genes responsible for some diseases and predict the chances of each of a couple's offspring having that disease; for others, it is only known that multiple hereditary and other factors play various roles in their occurrence. Environmental, social, occupational, and other influences may have significance equal to or greater than the hereditary.

Some genetic diseases or disorders can be seen immediately at or soon after birth, such as birth defects like a cleft lip or palate. Others, such as Huntington's chorea (the disease from which Woody Guthrie died), may take years to develop symptoms.

One classification of congenital or birth defects is those caused by a disorder in chromosomes. Chromosomes are the parts of cells that carry the genes that determine hereditary characteristics. Except for the sex cells (the egg and sperm), each cell has forty-six chromosomes found in twenty-three bonded pairs. Sex cells have twenty-three chromosomes, which join with the twenty-three of the mate to form a set of forty-six. Thus, your mother contributes half your chromosomes, your father the other half. Some newborns have extra chromosomes or lack a chromosome. In others, the structure or arrangement of the chromosomes is abnormal. Sometimes a chromosomal abnormality is the reason for an early miscarriage. Because each chromosome contains many genes, these disorders—called "syndromes"—affect many body systems and interfere with normal development. The best known is Down's syndrome (formerly called mongolism), which includes mental retardation.

We have included chromosomal disorders in this section because several show familial tendencies. Other nongenetic factors, however, may cause or contribute to their occurrence. These include X rays, before or during a pregnancy, drugs, chemical exposures, certain viruses, and parental age. Women over thirty-five are considered at risk for having a child with a chromosomal disorder, as are men over fifty-five. Down's syndrome, for example, appears in approximately one out of every thousand births among women less than thirty years old. At age thirty-five, the risk becomes one in 500, and it increases to one in 250 at age forty. If any of these disorders appears in your family's history, it is important to delve more deeply to uncover any of these other contributing agents.

There are a number of ways that disease can be directly inherited through genes. Five types of genetic inheritance are currently understood: dominant, recessive, mutation, sex-linked, and polygenic (or multifactorial).

For each inherited characteristic, such as eye color, you have two genes—one from each parent. You can receive the same or different genes from your two parents. If you receive two different genes, you will exhibit the dominant trait—in this example, brown eyes. The recessive trait—blue eyes—will show up only if you receive both genes for it. Blue-eyed people, therefore, must have two genes for blue eyes, and they can pass only that gene on to their offspring. So two blue-eyed parents cannot have a brown-eyed child. Two brown-eyed parents, however, can have a blue-eyed child if each of them was carrying a recessive gene for blue eyes and passed that gene on to their child.

Sickle-cell anemia is a recessive disease inherited in much the same way as blue eyes. Individuals with sickle-cell anemia must have two genes for the disease. A couple who both have sickle-cell anemia will always have children with the disease. If only one partner has the disease, each child will have that recessive gene; this is called sickle-cell trait. If a person with the trait reproduces with another person with the trait, their children may be normal (if they inherit two dominant, healthy genes), may have the trait (if they inherit only one recessive gene), or may have the disease (if they inherit a recessive gene from each parent). It is impossible to inherit sickle-cell anemia unless both parents have at least one recessive gene for it. Because you must inherit the same gene from both parents to exhibit such recessively inherited diseases, these may remain hidden in families for generations. Another example of a recessively inherited blood disease is thalessemia (or Cooley's anemia).

A number of metabolic disorders are also recessively inherited. In these, the affected person lacks a specific enzyme or hormone. Symptoms are usually multiple. These diseases include cystic fibrosis, phenylketonuria (PKU), hypothyroidism, and Tay-Sachs disease.

Examples of diseases inherited through dominant genes are Huntington's chorea and certain eye diseases such as retinitis pigmentosa and retinoblastoma.

Some inherited diseases appear originally as mutations. A mutation is a spontaneous change in a gene. This mechanism is responsible for achondroplasia—a type of dwarfism. Once this mutation occurs, achondroplasia is passed on as a dominant trait. This explains why, although somebody may be the first person in a family to have this disease, he or she can pass it on to his or her children.

Sex-linked traits are those whose genes are found on the female or X chromosome. All women have two X chromosomes while men have one X and one Y. Therefore, both males and females always inherit an X chromosome from their mother. If the egg cell is fertilized by a sperm carrying a Y chromosome, the resulting fetus will be male. If the sperm carries an X chromosome, the fetus will be female.

The vast majority of sex-linked diseases are carried or passed on by women, but rarely affect them. This is because most of these diseases (and nondisease traits, such as color blindness) are recessive characteristics. Because females need two diseased X chromosomes for the trait to appear, the only way for a woman to inherit most sex-linked diseases is if both her mother and father carry an affected gene—if her mother is a carrier and her father has the disease. This is extremely rare. A male, however, need only receive the gene from his mother on her X chromosome and he will exhibit the trait.

Women can pass an affected X chromosome to both sons and daughters—daughters will continue to be carriers; sons will be affected. A man can pass his X chromosome only to his daughter. Unless she also receives an affected X chromosome from her mother, she will be a carrier, not a sufferer. Since X-linked diseases are often quite serious, many of the men suffering from them never reproduce. Thus, the diseases are generally passed from mother to son, and the potential to carry the disease from mother to daughter. Hemophilia, the disease famous for having affected many European kings, is an example of a sex-linked disease. Duchenne's muscular dystrophy, a disabling and ultimately fatal illness, is a less-known sex-linked disease.

The category of polygenic or multifactorial inheritance encompasses many conditions. It includes diseases whose development depends on several genes and their particular combinations or on the combination of genetic and other causative agents such as chemicals, drugs, X rays, infections, medications, and life experiences. These diseases appear to have familiar tendencies but their patterns of occurrence do not correspond to patterns in which one gene is to blame. Your chances of having fraternal (nonlook-alike) twins is hereditary, but not related to one specific gene. Other examples include the many listed on the charts that follow.

We do not want to imply by this extensive list of familial diseases that heredity is the major cause of problems such as alcoholism, hypertension, or emotional disorders. Obviously, workplace and home stress and a multitude of knowns and unknowns contribute enormously to their development. Some illnesses listed, such as tuberculosis, require exposure to specific bacteria. This is not a hereditary factor, except insofar as people tend to live and work in the same environment as their relatives. Yet the tendency to develop the disease once exposure occurs seems to be familial.

In addition to inherited disease, we have included drugs taken by your mother during her pregnancy. It has recently been discovered that DES (diethylstilbestrol), a drug given in parts of the country to women in the 1940s, 1950s, and 1960s to prevent miscarriage, causes serious problems, including cancer, in their daughters and sons after ten or more years.* We have also provided space for you to include any less common illnesses among your relatives. We urge you to discuss with your health-care practitioner the possible significance of these to you and your family. Be especially alert to those that affect more than one family member.

We have included the age of onset and treatments received for each disease because these may provide clues to the seriousness of the disease and to the relative importance of the hereditary component in its transmission. Juvenile diabetes is, for example, less likely to be hereditary than is adult-onset diabetes. Diabetes that has to be treated with insulin injections may even be a different disease from diabetes controlled by diet. Finally, there is a place for you to record the place of birth and ethnicity of each close relative. This is because certain of the diseases listed occur primarily among specific populations. Tay-Sachs disease is found among Ashkenazic Jews (of Eastern European origin), sickle-cell anemia occurs among people of Mediterranean or African descent, and thalessemia is a disease of Italians, Greeks, and other Mediterranean people. If you discover that your ancestors came from these parts of the world, it may be advisable for you and your family members to have diagnostic tests for these illnesses.

---

* Researchers have not begun to investigate adequately the effects on a developing fetus of medications or other substances taken by a father prior to conception. For now, we have omitted this area, although in the future it may be found to be significant.

   Research is also insufficent on drugs and procedures used in modern-day obstetrics, such as Bendectin, a commonly prescribed antinausea drug, or ultrasound, a diagnostic test used almost routinely by some practitioners. See the section "Pregnancy" for charts that incorporate these data which will become the "family history" of your children.

We suggest that if you have never done so, you sit down with a close relative from each side of your family when you both have time. Record a thorough family health history. Your mate should do this as well, so that your children's family histories will be complete. We realize that this may be difficult for the many families in our country that are separated. Divorced, widowed, and single parents don't always have access to information about their mate's families. As with all areas of health maintenance and prevention, the gathering of a complete family history is a goal to be striven toward; it may not always be completely achievable.

Adoptive parents generally have no access to information about their children's biological parents. We recommend that when adopting a child, you submit these forms to the adoption agency. Explain your concern with your child's health, not as a prerequisite to adoption but as a health security measure for the child's future. Ask that the agency supply the information requested in these charts. If anonymity of parentage is the agency's policy, it can be maintained.

Bring your family health history with you when you consult a health-care practitioner for specific symptoms. Bring it with you to your first prenatal visit or to your child's first pediatric visit. Your practitioner will be impressed and appreciative. It will save time during the visit and allow you to discuss other concerns. It will help you receive complete, high-quality care, especially in the important areas of prevention and early detection of problems. These include the newly developed areas of genetic counseling and prenatal diagnosis.

For further information on genetics, genetic diseases, counseling, and prenatal diagnosis we suggest the following books:

> *Know Your Genes,* Aubrey Milunsky, Avon Books, 1979; Houghton Mifflin, 1977.
>
> *It's Not Too Late for a Baby: For Women and Men Over 35,* Sylvia Rubin, Prentice-Hall, Inc., 1980.
>
> *Birth Defects Compendium,* 2nd Edition, Daniel Bergsma, Editor, National Foundation—March of Dimes, Alan Liss, 1979.
>
> *Birth Defects and Drugs in Pregnancy,* O. P. Heinonen, Dennis Slone and Samuel Shapiro, Publishing Sciences Group, 1977.

FAMILY HISTORY

DISEASE OR DISORDER	RELATIVE(S)	AGE OF ONSET	TREATMENT(S)/ MEDICATION(S)/ OUTCOME
CHROMOSOMAL ABNORMALITIES Down's Syndrome			
Turner's Syndrome			
Klinefelter's Syndrome			
Other (specify)_______________			
HEREDITARY DISORDERS *Dominant Inheritance* Huntington's Chorea			
Marfan's Syndrome			
Retinitis Pigmentosa			
Retinoblastoma			
Recessive Inheritance Sickle-Cell Anemia trait			
Thalessemia			
Major (Cooley's Anemia)			
Minor			
Phenylketonuria (PKU)			
Tay-Sachs Disease			
Hypothyroidism			
Other Metabolic Disorders (specify)_______________			
Sex-Linked Inheritance Color Blindness			
Hemophilia			
Duchenne's Muscular Dystrophy			
Mental Retardation (some types)			
Hydrocephaly (some types)			

Name ________

Name

Mutations			
Achondrophasia (Dwarfism)			
Multifactorial Inheritance			
Birth Defects			
Cleft Lip/Palate			
Neural-Tube Defects (Anencephaly, Spina Bifida, Hydrocephaly)			
Congenital Heart Defects			
Limb Defects			
Other			
Diabetes			
Cancer (specify type)			
High Blood Pressure (Hypertension)			
Heart or Cardiovascular Disease (including stroke)			
Kidney (Renal) Problems			
Liver Disease			
Lung Disease (Asthma, Emphysema, Tuberculosis)			
Thyroid Disease			
Epilepsy (and other convulsive disorders)			
Allergies			
Migraine Headaches			
Glaucoma			
Cataracts			
Dyslexia (learning disorders)			
Obesity			
Crib Death (Sudden Infant Death Syndrome or SIDS)			
Psoriasis			

Multiple Sclerosis			
Myasthenia Gravis			
Hearing Disorders (some types)			
Multiple Pregnancies—twins, triplets, etc. (specify identical or fraternal)			
Systemic Lupus Erythematosis			
Nervous/Emotional Disorders			
Alcoholism			

Name

Name

NAME OF FAMILY MEMBER	PLACE OF BIRTH	ETHNICITY	OCCUPA-TION(S)	CAUSE OF DEATH	AGE AT DEATH	NOTES OR COMMENTS
MOTHER (note drugs taken during pregnancy with you)						
FATHER						
MOTHER'S MOTHER (Maternal Grandmother)						
MOTHER'S FATHER (Maternal Grandfather)						
FATHER'S MOTHER (Paternal Grandmother)						
FATHER'S FATHER (Paternal Grandfather)						
BROTHERS						
SISTERS						
CHILDREN						

FAMILY HISTORY

DISEASE OR DISORDER	RELATIVE(S)	AGE OF ONSET	TREATMENT(S)/ MEDICATION(S)/ OUTCOME
CHROMOSOMAL ABNORMALITIES Down's Syndrome			
Turner's Syndrome			
Klinefelter's Syndrome			
Other (specify)_______			
HEREDITARY DISORDERS *Dominant Inheritance* Huntington's Chorea			
Marfan's Syndrome			
Retinitis Pigmentosa			
Retinoblastoma			
Recessive Inheritance Sickle-Cell Anemia trait			
Thalessemia			
Major (Cooley's Anemia)			
Minor			
Phenylketonuria (PKU)			
Tay-Sachs Disease			
Hypothyroidism			
Other Metabolic Disorders (specify)_______			
Sex-Linked Inheritance Color Blindness			
Hemophilia			
Duchenne's Muscular Dystrophy			
Mental Retardation (some types)			
Hydrocephaly (some types)			

Name

Name

Mutations Achondrophasia (Dwarfism)			
Multifactorial Inheritance Birth Defects			
Cleft Lip/Palate			
Neural-Tube Defects (Anencephaly, Spina Bifida, Hydrocephaly)			
Congenital Heart Defects			
Limb Defects			
Other Diabetes			
Cancer (specify type)			
High Blood Pressure (Hypertension)			
Heart or Cardiovascular Disease (including stroke)			
Kidney (Renal) Problems			
Liver Disease			
Lung Disease (Asthma, Emphysema, Tuberculosis)			
Thyroid Disease			
Epilepsy (and other convulsive disorders)			
Allergies			
Migraine Headaches			
Glaucoma			
Cataracts			
Dyslexia (learning disorders)			
Obesity			
Crib Death (Sudden Infant Death Syndrome or SIDS)			
Psoriasis			

Multiple Sclerosis			
Myasthenia Gravis			
Hearing Disorders (some types)			
Multiple Pregnancies—twins, triplets, etc. (specify identical or fraternal)			
Systemic Lupus Erythematosis			
Nervous/Emotional Disorders			
Alcoholism			

Name

Name

NAME OF FAMILY MEMBER	PLACE OF BIRTH	ETHNICITY	OCCUPA-TION(S)	CAUSE OF DEATH	AGE AT DEATH	NOTES OR COMMENTS
MOTHER (note drugs taken during pregnancy with you)						
FATHER						
MOTHER'S MOTHER (Maternal Grandmother)						
MOTHER'S FATHER (Maternal Grandfather)						
FATHER'S MOTHER (Paternal Grandmother)						
FATHER'S FATHER (Paternal Grandfather)						
BROTHERS						
SISTERS						
CHILDREN						

NOTES

Medical History

Each of our medical histories tells the personal story of part of our past. Your goal in obtaining and sharing this information with your practitioner is to receive individualized and complete health care.

We have made this medical history quite comprehensive. It will take you back to your childhood, to all the places you've lived, and to each of your jobs.

Some childhood illnesses have consequences that extend into adulthood. An example of this is rheumatic fever, which can later result in heart problems. A person with a history of rheumatic fever may require medications to prevent heart infection during dental treatments, childbirth, or medical procedures.

Several childhood diseases are more serious if encountered as adults; these include German measles (rubella) during pregnancy and mumps in men. These, and some other viral illnesses, generally confer permanent immunity once contracted. It may be useful to be aware of which immunities have been gained in childhood and which not, to avoid exposure when necessary.

Remembering and recording where you've lived and worked, as well as the types of jobs you've held, may prove beneficial as more information is revealed on the potential dangers of environmental pollutants and chemicals used in industry. Most of us have heard of the tragic consequences of exposure of soldiers in Vietnam to "Agent Orange." Unfortunately, such dangers are not limited to warfare. It is not unlikely—bleak though the prospect may seem—that the future will bring more such exposés. They could involve any geographic area or workplace. Diagnostic tests, such as X rays, also carry risks. It is important to keep track of these to avoid a large buildup of exposure.

The amount of radiation in an X ray is measured in "rads," and this information should be available from a radiologist or X-ray technician.

Knowing about past and recent illnesses serves many purposes. Some viruses, such as herpes, never leave the body. Though symptoms subside and you feel well, these viruses may attack at any time, especially during periods of physical or emotional stress. Active genital herpes may be dangerous to an unborn child exposed during the birth process; your prenatal-care provider needs this information. Herpes may be associated with an increased risk of developing cervical cancer, so frequent Pap smears become necessary.

Some conditions, such as hypertension, are important to note because they increase the likelihood of your developing life-threatening diseases. Their existence in your medical history may signal the need for preventive measures such as dietary changes or exercise regimens. Others, such as anemia or phlebitis, add risks to surgery. Many conditions make certain medications inadvisable. It is also possible for two or more medications to have adverse affects when taken together. For this reason, we've left a place for you to include all current and past medication and drug use.

Knowledge of previous allergic reactions can be lifesaving. You may be the person who needs to carry an emergency insect-bite kit on hiking trips. You may be the patient who should never receive penicillin or other commonly prescribed medications. Since exposure to agents causing allergic responses (allergens) may be infrequent, it is easy to forget about such dangers. But such forgetfulness could endanger your life.

The results of important diagnostic tests should be a part of a medical history. This information may become important at a later date to prevent repetition of potentially dangerous tests. It also facilitates evaluation of the progress of a specific problem or disease through comparisons over time.

In each section of your medical history, we have asked for hospital and practitioner names and addresses. This is so that detailed data can be sent for if necessary at any time.

We have included sexual difficulties as part of this routine medical history. Perhaps some of you may not want to record these problems. We believe that sexual difficulties should not lead to silent suffering. It is unlikely that your problem is unique. Many sexual dysfunctions have their basis in a physical disorder; others come from emotional difficulties, and still others from a lack of bodily awareness and understanding. Help is available in each of these areas.

It is possible that your practitioner may be unprepared to deal with sexuality. Medical education does not necessarily teach treatments for sexual dysfunctions. A provider's personality may make support and counseling difficult. He or she should, however, know where to refer you. There are counselors whose specific area of expertise is sexuality. They work in both private practice and clinic settings. If your practitioner does not have this information, then your inquiries may lead to the development of an appropriate referral system.

As with some of the issues in the section "Discussing the 'Unspeakable,'" it may take some courage to raise sexual concerns, especially with a practitioner who seems impersonal or oriented to the technical. Open discussion may be the only way for you to receive help. Your openness may also sensitize your practitioner to such needs. This will surely benefit future patients.

Practitioners should always ask for a thorough medical history on your first visit with them or their clinic. Sometimes, their haste or your nervousness causes you to forget important facts or to omit significant details. This is understandable. We suggest that you do not wait for a health-care visit to complete this form. Do it at your leisure; it may require discussions with your parents or other older relatives who remember your childhood bouts with illness better than you do. Be as complete as possible.

Bring this chart with you when you seek the services of a new practitioner or are seen for the first time in a hospital or clinic. Some practitioners may want to look at the chart; most will still ask questions about your history. Your answers will be more precise and complete if you refer to this written history.

The material in the Occupational and Residential History charts was drawn from a questionnaire developed by Velma Campbell, M.D. We thank her for allowing us to use it.

HISTORY OF MEDICAL ILLNESSES

ILLNESS	DATE(S)	TREATMENT RECEIVED
Birth Defects (congenital anomalies) Specify_______________________		
Anemia Pernicious Anemia		
Iron-Deficiency Anemia		
Folic-Acid Deficiency		
Sickle-cell Anemia		
Sickle-cell Trait		
Thalessemia Major or Minor (specify)_______________		
Other (specify)_______________		
Other Blood Diseases (specify)_______		
Diabetes Mellitus		
Diabetes Insipidus		
Cancer (specify type)_______________		
High Blood Pressure (Hypertension) (specify usual levels)_______________		
Lung Disease (specify)_______________		
Rheumatic Fever		
Stomach or Intestinal Problems (gastrointestinal disease)		
Kidney Disease (renal disease)		
Urinary Tract Disease (such as bladder infections—cystitis, urethritis)		
Liver Disease (hepatitis, other— specify)_______________		
Infertility		
Phlebitis, varicose veins		
Convulsive Disorders (seizures, epilepsy—specify)_______________		
Nervous/Emotional Disorders		
Diseases of the Eye (specify)_______		
Diseases of the Ear (specify)_______		

Name

Name

Diseases of the Nose, Throat (specify)______________		
Thyroid Malfunctions (hyper- or hypothyroid, specify)______________		
Arthritis/Bursitis (specify)___________		
Accidents (specify)___________		
Other (specify)___________		
FOR WOMEN ONLY		
Vaginal Infections—Monilia (yeast, Candida)		
Cervicitis		
Sexually Transmitted Diseases—Vaginal Infections:		
Trichomonas		
Bacterial (Hemophilus, sometimes called nonspecific vaginitis)		
Chlamydia (may be without symptoms in women)		
Genital Warts (condylomata acuminata)		
Genital Herpes		
Syphilis		
Gonorrhea		
Pelvic Inflammatory Disease		
Bartholin's Gland Cyst		
Ovarian Cyst (specify left or right)		
Fibroid Uterus		
Sexual Disorders in Women:		
Inability to have orgasm primary (never had orgasm)		
secondary (has had orgasm)		
Lack of lubrication		
Painful intercourse (dyspareunia)		
Vaginismus (involuntary closing of vaginal muscles)		
Other (specify)___________		

FOR MEN ONLY		
Problems Involving Testicles (specify) ______________________		
Prostate Problems		
Sexually Transmitted Diseases:		
Trichomonas (without symptoms in men; must be treated if partner has symptoms)		
Hemophilus		
Nonspecific Urethritis (chlamydia)		
Genital Warts (condylomata acuminata)		
Genital Herpes		
Syphilis		
Gonorrhea		
Sexual Disorders in Men:		
Impotence primary (never had erection)		
secondary (has had erection)		
Premature ejaculation		
Other (specify) __________		

Name ________

RECORD OF HOSPITALIZATIONS
(List all hospitalizations, including during childhood)

REASON FOR HOSPITALIZATION	HOSPITAL NAME AND ADDRESS	PRACTITIONER NAME AND ADDRESS	DATE ADMITTED	DATE DISCHARGED

Name

OTHER SURGERIES

REASON	TYPE OF SURGERY	DATE	PRACTITIONER	LOCATION	EFFECTS

OTHER TREATMENTS
(Include chiropractic treatments, psychiatric treatments, acupuncture, special courses of treatment such as chemotherapy or radiation therapy, etc.)

TREATMENT	PRACTITIONER NAME AND ADDRESS	REASON	DATE(S)	RESULTS

RECORD OF HOSPITALIZATIONS (continued)
(For pregnancy and complications of pregnancy, see "Obstetrical History," p. 152)

SURGERY	OTHER TREATMENTS	MEDICATIONS	REACTIONS/RESULTS

OTHER DIAGNOSTIC TESTS
(See p. 91 for list of common diagnostic tests)

TEST	DATE	REASON	PRACTITIONER	HOSPITAL/OFFICE	RESULT

RECORD OF X RAYS

REASON	DATE	AREA X-RAYED AND NUMBER OF EXPOSURES AND RADS *(Ask radiologist or technician)*	DIAGNOSIS/ RESULT	HOSPITAL OR PRACTITIONER NAME AND ADDRESS

Name

CHILDHOOD ILLNESSES

ILLNESS	DATE(S)	SPECIAL TREATMENT (IF ANY)	LONG-TERM EFFECTS (IF ANY)
Measles (rubeola)			
Roseola			
Mumps			
German Measles (rubella)			
Chicken Pox (varicella)			
Mononucleosis			
Rheumatic Fever			
Scarlet Fever			
Tonsillitis _______			
_______			
Other (specify) _______			
_______			
_______			
_______			

Name

IMMUNIZATIONS

IMMUNIZATION/TYPE OF VACCINE	DATE(S)	IMMUNIZATION/TYPE OF VACCINE	DATE(S)
Measles (rubeola)		Diphtheria	
Mumps			
German Measles (rubella)			
Polio			
Type of vaccine _______		Tetanus	
How given: by mouth _______			
by injection _______			
		booster _______	
Smallpox		booster _______	
Other (specify) _______		booster _______	
_______			
_______			

TUBERCULOSIS SKIN TESTS

PPD OR TINE (SPECIFY)	DATE	RESULTS

RECORD OF ALLERGIES

(For more information on allergies, see p. 278 in section covering childhood)

TYPE OF ALLERGEN	NAME OF ALLERGEN	DATE OF REACTION	TYPE OF REACTION	TREATMENT AND RESULTS
DRUGS				
FOODS				
ANIMALS/INSECTS				
PLANTS				
OTHER				

Name

MEDICATION HISTORY
(Include prescribed and self-prescribed medications. Include herbal treatments and all drugs taken.)

DATE(S)	BRAND NAME	GENERIC NAME	REASON	DOSAGE	REACTIONS

Name

HISTORY OF HABITS AND LIFE-STYLE

Alcohol Use (List separately the periods of your life where alcohol consumption varied significantly)

TYPE	AMOUNT (PER DAY OR PER WEEK)	APPROXIMATE MONTHS OR YEARS USED

Narcotic, Barbiturate, and Tranquilizer Use (Include sleeping pills, Valium, "downers." Describe as for alcohol, above.)

DRUG	DOSAGE OR AMOUNT	APPROXIMATE MONTHS OR YEARS USED

Tobacco Use (Specify if pipe, cigars, chewing, cigarettes.)

TYPE	AMOUNT	NUMBER OF YEARS USED

COFFEE AND TEA DRINKING＿＿＿＿＿＿＿＿   Amount＿＿＿＿＿＿＿＿＿＿＿＿＿＿＿

BOWEL HABITS＿＿＿＿＿＿＿＿＿＿＿＿＿＿＿＿＿＿＿＿＿＿＿＿＿＿＿＿＿＿＿

BLADDER HABITS＿＿＿＿＿＿＿＿＿＿＿＿＿＿＿＿＿＿＿＿＿＿＿＿＿＿＿＿＿

HOBBIES

Materials Used

Name

OCCUPATIONAL HISTORY

DATES EMPLOYED		EMPLOYER NAME, ADDRESS, AND DEPARTMENT	TITLE OR JOB DESCRIPTION	HOURS/ SHIFTS WORKED	ON-JOB INJURIES	PROTECTIVE EQUIPMENT USED
FROM	TO					

RESIDENTIAL AND ENVIRONMENTAL HISTORY

Date of Birth _______________________________

City and State of Birth _______________________________

DATES OF RESIDENCE		STREET AND APARTMENT NUMBER	CITY AND STATE
FROM	TO		

OCCUPATIONAL HISTORY (continued)

EXTREME HEAT OR COLD	GASES (LIST TYPES)	NOISE LEVEL (DESCRIBE)	DUST (SPECIFY TYPE)	RADI-ATION	VIBRA-TION	LIST ALL CHEMICAL EXPOSURES

RESIDENTIAL AND ENVIRONMENTAL HISTORY (continued)

Hospital where born _______________

Practitioner attending birth _______________

WATER SOURCES (BOTTLE, WELL, NAME OF RIVER, ETC.)	PEST CONTROL (WHO PROVIDED: LIST BRAND NAMES IF KNOWN)	ENVIRONMENTAL NOTES (NEARBY INDUSTRY, HAZARDS, ETC.)

Name

MILITARY SERVICE HISTORY

Name

Branch of Service _______________ Dates _______ to _______

Describe all work performed _______________________________________

Where stationed _______________ Dates _______________ to _______

Combat duty (location) _______________ Dates _______________ to _______

Service-related injuries or disabilities:

Problem _______________ Date _______________ Treatment _______________

EXPOSURES TO HAZARDOUS SUBSTANCES	**DURATION OF EXPOSURE**	
List all chemical exposures, including defoliants and other chemical and biological warfare agents. List all radiation exposures, including handling of nuclear materials.	**FROM**	**TO**

PARTICIPATION IN EXPERIMENTS OR TESTS DURING MILITARY SERVICE

DATE	LOCATION	NATURE OF TEST OR EXPERIMENT	INDIVIDUAL ROLE/ PARTICIPATION	TEST RESULTS	SIDE EFFECTS

HISTORY OF MEDICAL ILLNESSES

ILLNESS	DATE(S)	TREATMENT RECEIVED
Birth Defects (congenital anomalies) Specify_______________________		
Anemia Pernicious Anemia		
Iron-Deficiency Anemia		
Folic-Acid Deficiency		
Sickle-cell Anemia		
Sickle-cell Trait		
Thalessemia Major or Minor (specify)_______________		
Other (specify)_______________		
Other Blood Diseases (specify)_______		
Diabetes Mellitus		
Diabetes Insipidus		
Cancer (specify type)_______________		
High Blood Pressure (Hypertension) (specify usual levels)_______________		
Lung Disease (specify)_______________		
Rheumatic Fever		
Stomach or Intestinal Problems (gastrointestinal disease)		
Kidney Disease (renal disease)		
Urinary Tract Disease (such as bladder infections—cystitis, urethritis)		
Liver Disease (hepatitis, other— specify)_______________		
Infertility		
Phlebitis, varicose veins		
Convulsive Disorders (seizures, epilepsy—specify)_______________		
Nervous/Emotional Disorders		
Diseases of the Eye (specify)_______		
Diseases of the Ear (specify)_______		

Name

Name

Diseases of the Nose, Throat (specify)_____________		
Thyroid Malfunctions (hyper- or hypothyroid, specify)_____________		
Arthritis/Bursitis (specify)_____________		
Accidents (specify)_____________		
Other (specify)_____________		
FOR WOMEN ONLY		
Vaginal Infections—Monilia (yeast, Candida)		
Cervicitis		
Sexually Transmitted Diseases—Vaginal Infections:		
Trichomonas		
Bacterial (Hemophilus, sometimes called nonspecific vaginitis)		
Chlamydia (may be without symptoms in women)		
Genital Warts (condylomata acuminata)		
Genital Herpes		
Syphilis		
Gonorrhea		
Pelvic Inflammatory Disease		
Bartholin's Gland Cyst		
Ovarian Cyst (specify left or right)		
Fibroid Uterus		
Sexual Disorders in Women:		
Inability to have orgasm primary (never had orgasm)		
secondary (has had orgasm)		
Lack of lubrication		
Painful intercourse (dyspareunia)		
Vaginismus (involuntary closing of vaginal muscles)		
Other (specify)_____________		

FOR MEN ONLY		
Problems Involving Testicles (specify) ________________		
Prostate Problems		
Sexually Transmitted Diseases:		
Trichomonas (without symptoms in men; must be treated if partner has symptoms)		
Hemophilus		
Nonspecific Urethritis (chlamydia)		
Genital Warts (condylomata acuminata)		
Genital Herpes		
Syphilis		
Gonorrhea		
Sexual Disorders in Men:		
Impotence primary (never had erection)		
secondary (has had erection)		
Premature ejaculation		
Other (specify)____________		

Name ________

RECORD OF HOSPITALIZATIONS
(List all hospitalizations, including during childhood)

REASON FOR HOSPITALIZATION	HOSPITAL NAME AND ADDRESS	PRACTITIONER NAME AND ADDRESS	DATE ADMITTED	DATE DISCHARGED

Name

OTHER SURGERIES

REASON	TYPE OF SURGERY	DATE	PRACTITIONER	LOCATION	EFFECTS

OTHER TREATMENTS
(Include chiropractic treatments, psychiatric treatments, acupuncture, special courses of treatment such as chemotherapy or radiation therapy, etc.)

TREATMENT	PRACTITIONER NAME AND ADDRESS	REASON	DATE(S)	RESULTS

RECORD OF HOSPITALIZATIONS *(continued)*
(For pregnancy and complications of pregnancy, see "Obstetrical History," p. 152)

SURGERY	OTHER TREATMENTS	MEDICATIONS	REACTIONS/RESULTS

OTHER DIAGNOSTIC TESTS
(See p. 91 for list of common diagnostic tests)

TEST	DATE	REASON	PRACTITIONER	HOSPITAL/OFFICE	RESULT

RECORD OF X RAYS

REASON	DATE	AREA X-RAYED AND NUMBER OF EXPOSURES AND RADS *(Ask radiologist or technician)*	DIAGNOSIS/ RESULT	HOSPITAL OR PRACTITIONER NAME AND ADDRESS

Name

CHILDHOOD ILLNESSES

Name

ILLNESS	DATE(S)	SPECIAL TREATMENT (IF ANY)	LONG-TERM EFFECTS (IF ANY)
Measles (rubeola)			
Roseola			
Mumps			
German Measles (rubella)			
Chicken Pox (varicella)			
Mononucleosis			
Rheumatic Fever			
Scarlet Fever			
Tonsillitis_______			
_______			
Other (specify) _______			
_______			
_______			

IMMUNIZATIONS

IMMUNIZATION/TYPE OF VACCINE	DATE(S)	IMMUNIZATION/TYPE OF VACCINE	DATE(S)
Measles (rubeola)		Diphtheria	
Mumps			
German Measles (rubella)			
Polio			
Type of vaccine_______		Tetanus	
How given: by mouth_______			
by injection_______			
		booster	
Smallpox		booster	
Other (specify)_______		booster	
_______			
_______			

TUBERCULOSIS SKIN TESTS

PPD OR TINE (SPECIFY)	DATE	RESULTS

RECORD OF ALLERGIES
(For more information on allergies, see p. 278 in section covering childhood)

TYPE OF ALLERGEN	NAME OF ALLERGEN	DATE OF REACTION	TYPE OF REACTION	TREATMENT AND RESULTS
DRUGS				
FOODS				
ANIMALS/INSECTS				
PLANTS				
OTHER				

Name

MEDICATION HISTORY
(Include prescribed and self-prescribed medications. Include herbal treatments and all drugs taken.)

Name

DATE(S)	BRAND NAME	GENERIC NAME	REASON	DOSAGE	REACTIONS
DATE(S)	BRAND NAME	GENERIC NAME	REASON	DOSAGE	REACTIONS

HISTORY OF HABITS AND LIFE-STYLE

Alcohol Use (List separately the periods of your life where alcohol consumption varied significantly)

TYPE	AMOUNT (PER DAY OR PER WEEK)	APPROXIMATE MONTHS OR YEARS USED

Narcotic, Barbiturate, and Tranquilizer Use (Include sleeping pills, Valium, "downers." Describe as for alcohol, above.)

DRUG	DOSAGE OR AMOUNT	APPROXIMATE MONTHS OR YEARS USED

Tobacco Use (Specify if pipe, cigars, chewing, cigarettes.)

TYPE	AMOUNT	NUMBER OF YEARS USED

COFFEE AND TEA DRINKING_______________   Amount_______________________

BOWEL HABITS____

BLADDER HABITS____

HOBBIES

Materials Used

OCCUPATIONAL HISTORY

DATES EMPLOYED		EMPLOYER NAME, ADDRESS, AND DEPARTMENT	TITLE OR JOB DESCRIPTION	HOURS/ SHIFTS WORKED	ON-JOB INJURIES	PROTECTIVE EQUIPMENT USED
FROM	TO					

RESIDENTIAL AND ENVIRONMENTAL HISTORY

Date of Birth____

City and State of Birth_______________________________________

DATES OF RESIDENCE		STREET AND APARTMENT NUMBER	CITY AND STATE
FROM	TO		

Name

OCCUPATIONAL HISTORY (continued)

EXTREME HEAT OR COLD	GASES (LIST TYPES)	NOISE LEVEL (DESCRIBE)	DUST (SPECIFY TYPE)	RADI-ATION	VIBRA-TION	LIST ALL CHEMICAL EXPOSURES

RESIDENTIAL AND ENVIRONMENTAL HISTORY (continued)

Hospital where born____

Practitioner attending birth____

WATER SOURCES (BOTTLE, WELL, NAME OF RIVER, ETC.)	PEST CONTROL (WHO PROVIDED: LIST BRAND NAMES IF KNOWN)	ENVIRONMENTAL NOTES (NEARBY INDUSTRY, HAZARDS, ETC.)

Name

MILITARY SERVICE HISTORY

Branch of Service _______________ Dates _______ to _______

Describe all work performed _____________________________________

Where stationed _________________ Dates _____________ to _________

Combat duty (location) ____________ Dates _____________ to _________

Service-related injuries or disabilities:

Problem _____________ Date _____________ Treatment _____________

EXPOSURES TO HAZARDOUS SUBSTANCES

List all chemical exposures, including defoliants and other chemical and biological warfare agents. List all radiation exposures, including handling of nuclear materials.

DURATION OF EXPOSURE

FROM	TO

PARTICIPATION IN EXPERIMENTS OR TESTS DURING MILITARY SERVICE

DATE	LOCATION	NATURE OF TEST OR EXPERIMENT	INDIVIDUAL ROLE/ PARTICIPATION	TEST RESULTS	SIDE EFFECTS

Practitioner Visits and Hospitalizations

As our society places increasing value on the achievement of health, the number of individuals involved in both health maintenance and curing of disease continues to expand. Paralleling the rise in numbers has been the rise in diversity and specialization of health workers.

The rapid growth in available knowledge and required technical skills has made this an inevitable trend. As we seek services, especially when we are sick or in need of help, we find ourselves confronted with a confusing maze of practitioners. Where to turn can be a difficult decision. If we have multiple problems, our confusion multiplies as well. We can easily feel fragmented; a different health practitioner may treat each separate problem until we wonder whether anyone remembers the whole person.

One solution to fragmentation is the "primary-care" provider. This physician or nurse-practitioner gives general-health care services for most of the problems we normally encounter. Many such physicians and nurse-practitioners provide care for all family members. When a difficulty arises that requires the attention of a specialist, the primary-care provider makes appropriate referrals and coordinates all aspects of care.

Specialization, however, need not lead to depersonalization. One way to avoid this is to assume an active role in your own care. Consider your practitioner a participant with you. Read as much as you can about health. Learn to develop opinions and discuss them with your practitioners. Don't be afraid to seek a second opinion, to discuss dissatisfaction about health care, or to change providers or clinics if you are unsatisfied with your care.

We realize that total choice is not always possible, especially for those dependent on municipal institutions and government funding for health services. We are also aware that not all practitioners welcome inquisitiveness on the part of patients. Some may seek increased power by withholding information. Others are simply not warm individuals. Still others mean well but become so involved in scientific intricacies that they lose sight of the human needs of their patients. Finally, years of intense and exhausting medical education sometimes leave scars, difficult to remove.

At times, it is not the practitioner who creates the relationship of inequality. We bring with us expectations of what a practitioner should be and should do. We often want to be relieved of self-responsibility. We seek miracle cures that require little or no effort on our part. We expect a parental, authoritarian figure in our practitioner and so we act childlike.

If these expectations and behaviors sound familiar to you, do not be surprised or blame yourself. Our society certainly glorifies members of the medical profession and instills feelings of awe toward them. Doctors make more money and have more prestige than almost anyone else. They limit the numbers entering the profession and accept mostly male members of the white middle and upper classes.

One large group that has become particularly conscious of its treatment by the medical profession has been women. As the women's movement emerged in the 1970s, it focused on, among other issues, health care. Women use health practitioners not only when they are sick but also for family planning, pregnancy, and postpartum care. As mothers, they use extensive well- and sick-child services. The women's movement questioned and denounced what it saw as patronizing practices, such as prescribing medications without full disclosure of their potential dangers. Women began to visit practitioners armed with written lists of questions. They went to see doctors in twos and threes to give each other support. And they formed self-help groups, reducing their reliance on the professional.

The pages that follow are designed to increase your participation in the aspects of your health care that require professional consultation. They provide space for you to write questions to ask your practitioner. Do this before each visit. When you are hospitalized, include questions for the various health-team members you encounter. The charts include columns for the results of tests taken and for treatments given. Just by recording these essentials, you will have increased your involvement in your care.

Always remember to inform your practitioners of other health care you are receiving. Tell them the names of medications you take. If you are pregnant, or think you might be, make sure they know this. Let them know, too, if you are breast-feeding. Each of these circumstances may affect your care.

We've divided practitioner visits into three sections. The first is for most health care. This includes visits to a variety of specialists such as family practitioner, gynecologist or nurse-midwife, physical therapist, or others you see on either a regular or an infrequent basis. Hospitalizations can be recorded on this chart, although prolonged hospital stays may require additional record-keeping in a separate notebook. We've made separate lists for dental and eye-care visits, since prevention in these two areas requires yearly checkups. Use and expand these charts as your personal needs require.

PRACTITIONER VISITS AND HOSPITALIZATIONS

DATE	NAME, ADDRESS, AND TITLE OF PRACTITIONER/ NAME AND ADDRESS OF HOSPITAL	REASON FOR VISIT (CHECKUP, OR LIST SYMPTOMS)	QUESTIONS TO ASK PRACTITIONER(S)	WEIGHT	BLOOD PRES- SURE	OTHER TESTS (PAP SMEAR, BLOOD TEST)

Name

TEST RESULTS	PRACTITIONER'S DIAGNOSIS	TREATMENTS/MEDICATIONS			INSTRUCTIONS	REFERRALS	SIDE EFFECTS NOTED
		NAME	HOW OFTEN	WITH/ BETWEEN MEALS			

Name

PRACTITIONER VISITS AND HOSPITALIZATIONS

DATE	NAME, ADDRESS, AND TITLE OF PRACTITIONER/ NAME AND ADDRESS OF HOSPITAL	REASON FOR VISIT (CHECKUP, OR LIST SYMPTOMS)	QUESTIONS TO ASK PRACTITIONER(S)	WEIGHT	BLOOD PRES- SURE	OTHER TESTS (PAP SMEAR, BLOOD TEST)

Name _______

TEST RESULTS	PRACTITIONER'S DIAGNOSIS	TREATMENTS/MEDICATIONS			INSTRUCTIONS	REFERRALS	SIDE EFFECTS NOTED
		NAME	HOW OFTEN	WITH/ BETWEEN MEALS			

Name

EYE-CARE VISITS

DATE	NAME AND ADDRESS OPTOMETRIST/ OPHTHALMOLOGIST	REASON FOR VISIT (E.G., YEARLY CHECK, BLURRY VISION, ETC.)	QUESTIONS TO ASK
DATE	NAME AND ADDRESS OPTOMETRIST/ OPHTHALMOLOGIST	REASON FOR VISIT (E.G., YEARLY CHECK, BLURRY VISION, ETC.)	QUESTIONS TO ASK

Name

RESULTS OF EYE EXAM	TREATMENTS (SUCH AS EYEGLASSES, MEDICATIONS, EXERCISES)	REFERRALS	SPECIAL INSTRUCTIONS

Name

DENTAL VISITS

Name

DATE	NAME AND ADDRESS OF PRACTITIONER	REASON FOR VISIT (E.G., CHECKUP, TOOTHACHE, BLEEDING GUMS, ETC.)	QUESTIONS TO ASK	NO. OF X RAYS	ABDOMINAL SHIELD USED?

TREATMENTS/MEDICATIONS/ ANESTHESIA (E.G., FILLINGS, EXTRACTIONS, NITROUS OXIDE, ETC.)	POST-TREATMENT MEDICATIONS			REACTIONS NOTED	SPECIAL REFERRALS/ INSTRUCTIONS
	NAME	HOW OFTEN	SPECIAL INSTRUC- TIONS		

Name

PRACTITIONER VISITS AND HOSPITALIZATIONS

Name _______________

DATE	NAME, ADDRESS, AND TITLE OF PRACTITIONER/ NAME AND ADDRESS OF HOSPITAL	REASON FOR VISIT (CHECKUP, OR LIST SYMPTOMS)	QUESTIONS TO ASK PRACTITIONER(S)	WEIGHT	BLOOD PRES-SURE	OTHER TESTS (PAP SMEAR, BLOOD TEST)

TEST RESULTS	PRACTITIONER'S DIAGNOSIS	TREATMENTS/MEDICATIONS			INSTRUCTIONS	REFERRALS	SIDE EFFECTS NOTED
		NAME	HOW OFTEN	WITH/ BETWEEN MEALS			

Name

PRACTITIONER VISITS AND HOSPITALIZATIONS

Name ________

DATE	NAME, ADDRESS, AND TITLE OF PRACTITIONER/ NAME AND ADDRESS OF HOSPITAL	REASON FOR VISIT (CHECKUP, OR LIST SYMPTOMS)	QUESTIONS TO ASK PRACTITIONER(S)	WEIGHT	BLOOD PRES-SURE	OTHER TESTS (PAP SMEAR, BLOOD TEST)

TEST RESULTS	PRACTITIONER'S DIAGNOSIS	TREATMENTS/MEDICATIONS			INSTRUCTIONS	REFERRALS	SIDE EFFECTS NOTED
		NAME	HOW OFTEN	WITH/ BETWEEN MEALS			

Name

EYE-CARE VISITS

Name

DATE	NAME AND ADDRESS OPTOMETRIST/ OPHTHALMOLOGIST	REASON FOR VISIT (E.G., YEARLY CHECK, BLURRY VISION, ETC.)	QUESTIONS TO ASK
DATE	NAME AND ADDRESS OPTOMETRIST/ OPHTHALMOLOGIST	REASON FOR VISIT (E.G., YEARLY CHECK, BLURRY VISION, ETC.)	QUESTIONS TO ASK

RESULTS OF EYE EXAM	TREATMENTS (SUCH AS EYEGLASSES, MEDICATIONS, EXERCISES)	REFERRALS	SPECIAL INSTRUCTIONS

Name

DENTAL VISITS

Name ___________

DATE	NAME AND ADDRESS OF PRACTITIONER	REASON FOR VISIT (E.G., CHECKUP, TOOTHACHE, BLEEDING GUMS, ETC.)	QUESTIONS TO ASK	NO. OF X RAYS	ABDOMINAL SHIELD USED?

TREATMENTS/MEDICATIONS/ ANESTHESIA (E.G., FILLINGS, EXTRACTIONS, NITROUS OXIDE, ETC.)	POST-TREATMENT MEDICATIONS			REACTIONS NOTED	SPECIAL REFERRALS/ INSTRUCTIONS
	NAME	HOW OFTEN	SPECIAL INSTRUC- TIONS		

Name

LISTS OF PRACTITIONERS

To help you understand the various categories of health workers and to choose appropriate practitioners for each of your family's needs, we have prepared this list of health specialists. We have included only those practitioners who deal directly with people; we've omitted "behind-the-scenes" workers who staff medical laboratories, design and conduct research programs, read and interpret diagnostic tests, answer phones and carry messages, build and repair medical equipment, maintain cleanliness of facilities, sterilize equipment, and perform a myriad of other essential services.

We have divided this list into three types of practitioners—medical, dental, and health practitioners. The first group is the doctors, those who've graduated from medical or osteopathic school and then have specialized in the fields listed. The second group consists of graduates of dental schools; they are also called "Doctor." The third group includes a variety of practitioners with many different educational backgrounds. Many of these health practitioners hold doctoral degrees and rightly call themselves "Doctor," sometimes creating confusion in our minds. Their degrees are not "M.D." degrees, however. They may have chiropractic degrees, optometric degrees, Ph.D. (Doctor of Philosophy) degrees, or others. Their educational backgrounds are not necessarily higher or lower than the M.D.'s, just different.

This list gives a brief definition or description of many types of health workers. We know that it is not complete; there are small numbers of highly specialized practitioners likely to have been left out. It does, however, give an idea of the great variety of health-care providers and what they do.

Medical Specialists

Physicians specialize by choosing age groups, body systems, diseases, or specific techniques as their area of expertise. New specialties and subspecialties arise frequently as knowledge becomes more sophisticated, life-styles change, and the environment and workplace become increasingly hazardous. Examples of new areas of medical expertise are occupational health, preventive medicine, emergency medicine, and sports medicine. Specialty education is provided after medical school through internship, residency, and fellowship programs. The length of these programs varies with the specialty. Certifying examinations are available in many of the specialties. Find out if your physician's specialty is a certified one and, if so, if he or she holds a certificate or has met the eligibility requirements for the examination.

The designation M.D. after a name means Doctor of Medicine. Other initials seen following M.D. may refer to the specialty organization to which the physician belongs (e.g., F.A.C.O.G. means Fellow of the American College of Obstetricians and Gynecologists). This implies certification. Other initials (e.g., P.C.) mean the practitioner is incorporated and do not refer at all to technical training, expertise, or degrees. Ask your practitioner what the initials following his name stand for and what that means.

NAME OF SPECIALTY OR SUB-SPECIALTY	*AREA OF SPECIALTY*
anesthesiologist	anesthesia
allergist	allergies
cardiologist	the heart and blood vessels (cardiovascular system)
dermatologist	the skin
endocrinologist	the glandular system and its hormones
family practitioner	comprehensive care to all family members. A better trained, modern "general practitioner." Is able to deal with the majority of problems and coordinate referrals to other specialists as needed
gastroenterologist	the stomach, intestines, and related digestive organs
general practitioner	similar to family practitioner, but has not completed a residency program
gerontologist	the aged
gynecologist	the female reproduction system (is usually also an obstetrician)
hematologist	the blood
hepatologist	the liver
hypnotist	hypnosis
immunologist	the immune system
infectious disease specialist	contagious diseases caused by various microorganisms
internist	adults
neonatologist	the newborn, especially the sick
neoplastic disease specialist	tumors
nephrologist	the kidneys
neurologist	the brain and nervous system
nuclear medical specialist	tests and treatments using radioactive substances
obstetrician	pregnancy
oncologist	cancers
ophthalmologist	the eyes
otorhinolaryngologist	the ears, nose, and throat (may be an otologist, rhinologist, or laryngologist)
orthopedist	the bones, joints, and muscles
pediatrician	children (may subspecialize in adolescents)
physiatrist	physical therapy
psychiatrist	the emotions
orthomolecular psychiatrist	nutrition and vitamins
pulmonary medical specialist	the lungs and respiratory system
radiologist	X rays and other radiation therapy
rheumatologist	diseases of the joints and connective tissues
surgeon	operative procedures—surgery (many subspecialties)
urologist	the urinary tract

Some physicians narrow their field of work even further. For example, a pediatrician can be a specialist in any of the body systems or organs mentioned. You find pediatric nephrologists and pediatric hematologists.

Surgeons often specialize in one type of surgery or one body system. There are plastic surgeons who do reconstructive work, cardiac surgeons who operate only on hearts, and neurosurgeons who work on the nervous system. There are various kinds of microsurgeons who use microscopes to perform delicate eye operations, reconnect limbs, and clear blocked Fallopian tubes to restore fertility in women.

The following practitioners attend educational programs separate from medical schools. Their practice, however, falls into the category of medicine.

NAME OF SPECIALTY	*AREA OF SPECIALTY*
Osteopath (D.O.)	comprehensive medical and surgical care with an emphasis on the musculoskeletal system
Podiatrist (D.P.M.)	complete medical and surgical care of the foot

Dental Practitioners (D.D.S. or D.M.D.)

Dentist	the teeth and related structures
Dental Surgeon (or Oral Surgeon)	operating on the teeth and mouth
Endodontist	prevention and treatment of diseases of the dental pulp and surrounding tissues
Orthodontist	prevention and correction of irregularities of the teeth
Pedodontist	children's teeth
Periodontist	diseases of tissues around the teeth (e.g., the gums)
Prosthodontist	making and fitting artificial teeth

Health Practitioners

We no longer think of health merely as the absence of disease or illness. Twentieth-century scientific understanding has widened our vision so that we rightfully desire a high level of health or wellness. As our demands increase for disease prevention, energetic living, relaxation, sexual satisfaction, and optimal functioning despite disease or disability, so do the numbers of people concerned with providing such services.

The following is an alphabetical listing of health specialists who provide direct services. We have included a wide range of practitioners—traditional and nontraditional. Their education and specific training varies, even within some of the specialties. Some areas of practice are licensed or certified; others are not regulated at all. Regulatory laws vary from state to state and change periodically within each state. When consulting a practitioner it is appropriate to ask whether the specialty is licensed or otherwise regulated within your state. If so, find out if your practitioner holds a license or certificate to practice.

New practitioners will undoubtedly arise as knowledge grows, technology advances, and our appreciation of the components of health expands.

Abused-Woman's Counselor: provides emotional and practical support for female victims of abuse.

Acupuncturist: administers the ancient Chinese science that uses needles for diagnosis, anesthesia, and healing.

Art Therapist: uses art as a form of therapy for physical and emotional problems.

Audiologist (C.C.A.): administers hearing tests and diagnoses and assesses hearing impairments. Corrects such impairments through the selection and fitting of hearing aids, training for speech reading, and referral to ear, nose, and throat physicians when necessary.

Biofeedback Therapist: works to enhance the ability to relax through the use of a machine that tells the subject when his or her body is in its most relaxed state.

Childbirth/Parent Educator (C.C.E.): teaches classes for pregnant women and their partners and for new parents.

Chiropractor (D.C.): manipulates the spine to correct disabilities.

Dance Therapist: uses dance as a form of therapy for emotional and physical problems.

Dental Hygienist: prevents diseases of the mouth through education about oral hygiene and by providing oral prophylactic care—cleaning of the teeth. May also assist with other dental tasks such as removing sutures, placing packs, and taking impressions.

EKG Technician: administers electrocardiograms (tests of the heart function).

Emergency Medical Technician (E.M.T.): works in ambulances. Provides on-the-spot care before and during transfer to a hospital. May be called a "paramedic."

Exercise Physiologist: designs and helps people implement exercise programs to maintain health and correct deficiencies.

Family-Planning Counselor: provides educational information and material about birth control. Dispenses methods available without a prescription—foam, suppositories, condoms.

Genetic Counselor: advises prospective parents on the probabilities of their passing on inherited diseases based on family histories and genetic profiles.

Herbalist: specializes in the use of naturally growing substances (herbs) as treatments and preventions.

Hypnotherapist: uses hypnosis for therapeutic purposes such as weight reduction and stopping smoking.

Masseur (Masseuse) or Massage Therapist: gives therapeutic massages. There are many types of massage including *shiatsu,* a Japanese pressure technique, Swedish massage, and rolfing, a deep muscle massage.

Medical Assistant: assists doctors in their offices in performing a variety of functions, including secretarial, nursing, and laboratory-related tasks.

Midwife: There are two kinds of midwives in this country:

    Empirical (or Practicing or Lay) Midwife: attends childbirths in the home. Provides prenatal care, labor and delivery services, and postpartum care.

Certified Nurse-Midwife (C.N.M.): provides prenatal services, labor and delivery care, postpartum, family-planning, and well-woman gynecologic services. Cares for the normal newborn. A certified nurse-midwife works in consultation with a physician but provides total, independent care for healthy women and their newborns. Works in the hospital, home, clinic, or birth center.

Music Therapist: uses music as a form of therapy for physical and emotional problems.

Nurse: There are two types of nurses in this country:

Licensed practical (or vocational) nurse (L.P.N. or L.V.N.): provides bedside care in homes and hospitals.

Registered nurse (R.N.): provides a broad spectrum of health-related care. Traditionally involved in the care of the sick, today's nurses also participate in health maintenance and health education. Nurses manage the totality of a patient's care and coordinate the various health-team members involved in that care. Supervise practical nurses and nurse's aides. An increasing number of nurses specialize in one area, providing highly skilled services. These include cardiac-care nurses, perinatal nurses, psychiatric nurses, gerontological nurses, orthopedic nurses, kidney-dialysis nurses, and numerous others.

Nurse-Anesthetist (C.N.A.): administers anesthesia.

Nurse-Practitioner (N.P.): performs physical examinations and diagnosis. Provides health-maintenance services and treats minor illnesses. Provides referrals to physicians as needed. May be an adult, pediatric, geriatric, or family nurse-practitioner (A.N.P., P.N.P., G.N.P., F.N.P.)

Nurse's Aide: a nursing assistant. Often provides much bedside care in hospitals. May do home care. Works under the supervision of a registered nurse.

Nutritionist (R.D.—Registered Dietician): provides educational services for all nutritional needs. Designs meal programs for special needs such as weight reduction, management of diabetes or heart disease, pregnancy and breast-feeding. Plans institutional dietary programs in a variety of settings.

Occupational Therapist (O.T.R.): aids disabled individuals to develop and maintain the ability to perform tasks and skills required in life.

Optometrist (O.D.): examines eyes and prescribes and fits corrective glasses and contact lenses. Designs therapeutic exercise programs. Screens for eye diseases and provides referrals to opthalmologists as necessary.

Physical Therapist (R.P.T.): designs and implements programs for rehabilitation and prevention of disability following disease, injury, or loss of body parts.

Physician's Assistant (P.A.): a physician extender. Performs physical examinations and diagnoses. Cares independently for minor illnesses, but always works with a physician. May be medical or surgical.

Psychologist (M.S., Ph.D.): provides emotional-counseling services for individuals and groups. Differs from a psychiatrist in education and in nonreliance on medications. A wide variety of schools of thought and orientations are found in psychology. Many psychologists specialize in one area such as marriage counseling, family therapy, or child psychology.

Rape Crisis Counselor: provides emotional and practical support for rape victims. Works on-call for immediate care and provides long-term follow-up to individuals and groups.

Recreational Therapist: uses recreational activities such as arts and crafts as a form of therapy for physical and emotional problems.

Respiratory Therapist (R.R.T.): administers therapies for respiratory problems. Cares for patients on breathing machines.

Sex Therapist: provides therapy for problems relating to sexual function and pleasure.

Social Worker (M.S.W. or C.S.W.): provides counseling services for people with social and emotional problems. Helps individuals and families "deal with the system." Can help people obtain welfare benefits, food stamps, and homemaker services, for example. Works in various agencies such as foster care services, hospitals, and senior citizen centers.

Sonographer: performs sonograms (sound-wave pictures) and interprets results.

Special Educator: provides basic education for children and adults with various disabilities such as deafness, blindness, a variety of learning disorders, and physical diseases such as cerebral palsy.

Speech Pathologist: corrects abnormalities in the making of sounds through diagnosis and training.

X-ray Technician or Radiologic Technologist: Assistant to a radiologist. Performs X rays and operates radiographic equipment.

COMMON DIAGNOSTIC TESTS

Record-keeping will make more sense to you if you understand tests that are done to diagnose possible health problems. The number of such tests available to practitioners is staggering, however. Every body fluid and discharge is subject to laboratory analysis. All body cavities can be examined. X rays, sonograms, and now CAT scans using computers allow any part of the body to be visualized. A complete list of diagnostic tests with even brief explanations could easily become another book. We have decided to list, instead, categories of those tests commonly used and give examples of some conditions they detect. Of course, the most basic diagnostic "tests" are a general history and physical examination.

See the section "Routine Tests and Examinations in Pregnancy" (p. 172) for descriptions of the following:

Complete blood count (CBC)	Sickle-cell screen
Urinalysis (U/A)	Blood type and Rh examinations
Pap smear	Tine or PPD tests for TB
Tests for gonorrhea and syphilis	Fasting blood sugar (FBS)
Rubella immunity screen	and 2-hour Postprandial (2 hr. PP)

See "Special Diagnostic Tests in Pregnancy" (p. 176) for:

Chest X ray (CXR)	Urine culture and sensitivity
Sonogram	Glucose tolerance test
Viral studies	Anemia work-up

All of the above tests apply to nonpregnant as well as to pregnant people. The section "Contraceptive History" (p. 140) notes the tests that need to be done for women using various types of contraceptives.

For healthy adults, the following tests should be repeated at intervals as screening for problems:

For women:
Pap smear: current American Cancer Society guidelines suggest a Pap Smear every three years following two negative tests taken one year apart if no other risk factors are present.
Breast exam: should be performed yearly by practitioners and monthly by yourself. See page 135 for a description of how to do a breast self-examination.

For women and men:
Blood pressure measurement
Skin test for tuberculosis
Urinalysis
Complete blood count
Serology (VDRL)
Blood chemistries (see below)
Eye test for vision
Dental examination for condition of the teeth and gums. May include X rays

For those over age 35:
Electrocardiogram (EKG)
Tonometry: test of the eye for glaucoma
Stool for occult (hidden) blood (also called "guiac")

For those over age 55:
Protoscopy: examination of the rectum for rectal cancer

Some specific tests for when you are having a problem include:

Blood tests
Blood chemistries:
   For example:
   SMA 6, SMA 12, liver function tests (LFTs), cholesterol, and tricyclerides:
   Analyses of the blood which measure levels of necessary chemicals. Provide information about health of many body systems and organs.
Clotting studies:
   For example:
   Platelets, prothrombin time (PT), partial thromboplastin time (PTT), Fibrinogen and clotting factors.
   Used to diagnose bleeding disorders.
Thyroid studies:
   For example:
   T_3 and T_4, resin uptake, TSH.
   Used to diagnose hypo- and hyperthyroid.

The following diseases are among those that can be diagnosed with blood tests:
   Hepatitis, mononucleosis, systemic lupus erythematus, various anemias, leukemia, syphilis.

To diagnose infections, the following blood tests might be done:
   Erythrocyte sedimentation rate (ESR): a special test of the red blood cells (RBCs).
   Differential: measures various types of white blood cells (WBCs) present in the blood.

Blood gas analyses:
>   Test blood in the arteries for pH (acidity), oxygen and carbon dioxide partial pressures to measure the ability of the lungs to maintain normal gas levels in the body. Used in respiratory disorders.

X rays:

X rays can visualize bones to determine fractures and dislocations. The amount of radiation in an X ray is measured in "rads."

Special X rays using dyes are used to visualize soft tissue which can't normally be seen on X rays. Examples of these are:
>   Upper G.I. series: to check the condition of the upper digestive tract. Helpful in diagnosing ulcers.
>   Cholecystogram: to study the gallbladder.
>   Barium enema: to assess the health of the intestines.
>   Intravenous pyelogram: to study the kidneys.

CAT (CTT) scan (Computerized Axial Tomography): a new computerized method of taking a series of X rays with low-dose radiation to give a three-dimensional picture of a part of the body.

Nuclear Medicine Scan:
>   A method of visualizing some structures of the body by injecting a small amount of radioactive substance which will selectively go to the part of the body to be scanned. This allows organs to be visualized using a machine similar to a Geiger counter.

Biopsies:
>   Laboratory analyses of a piece of tissue taken from an organ or a growth. Can test for cancer.

"Scopies":
>   A "Scopy" test involves the use of a special light to look into a body cavity and possibly a microscope to closely examine the condition of the tissues.
>   Examples include:
>   Culposcopy: looks through the vagina to the cervix. Done when a Pap smear is abnormal.
>   Proctoscopy: looks through the anus to visualize rectal tissue.
>   Bronchoscopy: looks at the bronchi, part of the upper respiratory tract.
>   Ophthalmoscopic exam: looks at the vessels of the eye grounds.

Cultures:
>   Tests in which a swab from one part of the body (e.g., the throat) or a sample of a body discharge (e.g., urine, sputum, pus) is sent to a lab to see if bacteria grow.

Sensitivities:
>   Determine which antibiotics can cure the specific bacteria found in a culture.

Tests of the Heart and Cardiovascular System:
>   Electrocardiogram (EKG or ECG): shows the pattern of electrical impulses in the heart.

Echocardiogram: A sonogram of the heart. Shows size of the chambers of the heart and valve functioning.

Cardiac catheterization: a test in which a tube is placed into an artery (usually in the groin) and passed through the chambers of the heart to measure pressure in the chambers and their blood flow.

Angiogram: uses a dye to study the heart and major blood vessels.

Tests of the Central Nervous System:

Spinal tap or lumbar puncture (LP): a sample of cerebrospinal fluid (CSF) is taken through the spinal canal. Can test for bacterial or viral infection, neurosyphilis, tuberculosis, multiple sclerosis, tumors, or hemorrhages.

Electroencephalogram (EEG): tests of the brain waves. Used for diagnosing convulsive and other neurological disorders.

Pulmonary Function Tests:

Test lung function. Used in respiratory problems such as emphysema, bronchitis, asthma.

Fertility Studies:

Many tests are done if a couple is unsuccessful in conceiving.

Examples include:

Sperm Count: for the male

Laparoscope: for a woman. A visualization of the Fallopian tubes through a small incision below the navel.

Hysterogram: An X-ray examination of the uterus with special dye to visualize its cavity.

24-hour urine collection: looks at levels of various hormones to study endocrine function.

Chromosomal Analysis (Karyotyping):

A method of looking at the chromosome pattern in a sample cell to study hereditary or congenital diseases.

NOTES

LONG-TERM ILLNESS

This book cannot provide space for those with long-term or chronic health problems to keep adequate records of health status, treatments, surgeries, dietary or exercise needs. If you wish to keep such a record, it might be convenient to keep a small notebook as a companion volume to this workbook. The following pages offer sample charts so that you can organize such a record. Naturally, you will have to adapt this to your individual needs.

Although more common in adults, long-term, chronic, or disabling illnesses do occur in children. This chart can be used for both the adult and child members of your family, as needed.

DIAGNOSIS AND PRACTITIONERS

Illness ____

Date Diagnosed _______________________________________

Physician Name ____

Address ____

____

Telephone ____

Other practitioners and services (for example, physical therapist, occupational therapist, social worker, psychologist, home health aide, Visiting Nurse Service)

NAME	SPECIALTY/SERVICE	ADDRESS	PHONE

SUPPORT AGENCIES

For example, American Cancer Society, American Diabetes Association, American Heart Association, Ostomy Clubs, Reach for Recovery

ORGANIZATION	INDIVIDUALS COUNSELORS OR CONTACTS	ADDRESS	PHONE

INITIAL DIAGNOSTIC TESTS

For example, glucose tolerance test, G.I. series (upper, lower), X rays, sonograms, CAT scans, etc. (See "Common Diagnostic Tests," p. 91)

TEST	DATE	RESULT	PRACTITIONER/HOSPITAL

OTHER INITIAL LABORATORY TESTS

For example, blood counts

TEST	DATE	RESULT	PRACTITIONER/HOSPITAL

HOME DIAGNOSTIC TESTS *(self-administered)*

For example, diabetic urine testing (This can be a large section)

TEST	EQUIPMENT NEEDED	SPECIAL INSTRUCTIONS	DATE	RESULT

Name

SYMPTOMS, FOLLOW-UP TESTS, AND TREATMENTS

DATE	SYMPTOM(S) NOTED	PRACTITIONER VISITED	LABORATORY TESTS AND RESULTS

Name

SPECIAL DIETS

To help maintain your special diet, you may choose to keep a written diary of what you eat. This can be done simply.

	MONDAY	TUESDAY	WEDNESDAY	THURSDAY	FRIDAY	SATURDAY	SUNDAY
BREAKFAST							
SNACK							
LUNCH							
SNACK							
DINNER							
SNACK							

You can make a checklist of the specific foods you must be certain to include each day and those foods you must avoid.

You can attach any diet instructions or plans provided by your practitioners.

See the section "Nutrition" (p. 100) for further dietary information.

SYMPTOMS, FOLLOW-UP TESTS, AND TREATMENTS (continued)

PRACTITIONER RECOMMENDATIONS AND INSTRUCTIONS	ACTIONS TAKEN AND NOTES

Name

ACTIVITY PLAN

Number of hours of rest needed per day _____________ Total exercise per day _____________

EXERCISE	NUMBER OF MINUTES/ HOURS PER DAY	NUMBER OF DAYS PER WEEK	SPECIAL EQUIPMENT NEEDED	PULSE BEFORE	RATE AFTER	SIDE EFFECTS NOTED OR SPECIAL INSTRUCTIONS

NUTRITION

In the late 1970s, both the Senate Committee on Nutrition and the Surgeon General of the United States called for significant changes in the typical American eating pattern. Their concern grew out of the knowledge that at least six major causes of death in this country have been identified as related to the way we eat: heart disease, hypertension and stroke, arteriosclerosis, diabetes, cirrhosis of the liver, and the following cancers—stomach, liver, small and large intestine, rectum, breast, uterus, prostate, and gallbladder.

The elements of food necessary for health are called nutrients. They are carbohydrates, proteins, vitamins, minerals, fats, and water. These categories are based on chemical composition and the role played in our bodies by each group of substances.

Carbohydrates consist of sugars (simple carbohydrates) and starches (complex carbohydrates). They provide us with energy.

Proteins are made up of amino acids. They are necessary for growth and repair of body tissues. In order for a protein food to be useful in the body it must contain all the amino acids that the body itself can't make—the eight "essential" amino acids. Such a protein is called a "complete" protein. Complete proteins are found in animal products. Plant sources of protein can be combined so that they provide complete proteins. For example, grains and beans together make a complete protein (rice and beans).

Vitamins are defined as substances essential for life. There are two types of vitamins—water-soluble and fat-soluble. The vitamins in the Vitamin B complex and Vitamin C are water-soluble. The body cannot store these, so daily intake is important. Vitamins A, D, E, and K are fat-soluble. Fats, therefore, are needed for the body to use these vitamins.

Fats also serve as a source of energy; fatty acids are necessary for growth. There are two kinds of fats. *Saturated* fats are solid at room temperature; these are found in animal products. *Unsaturated* fats are liquid at room temperature, with the exception of coconut oil and cocoa butter. These are found in plant products.

Water is the main chemical compound of our bodies. Without it, metabolic processes necessary for life could not occur. Human beings can exist for only short periods of time without water.

Minerals are inorganic elements or compounds, certain of which are necessary for life. The major body minerals are calcium, phosphorus, potassium, sodium, magnesium, sulfur, and chlorine. Examples of minerals found in smaller amounts (called trace minerals) are iron, copper, iodine, and zinc.

The specific dietary improvements proposed by the Senate and the Surgeon General include reducing our intake of sugar, salt, fat (especially saturated fat), and cholesterol, a substance found in the fat of animal products. Increasing the consumption of complex carbohydrates is recommended. Caloric intake should be limited to the amount actually used in daily activities—less for overweight people. In terms of actual foods eaten, these changes should mean more fruits, vegetables, and whole grains (complex carbohydrates); more fish, poultry, legumes (beans and peas); and fewer sweets and sweetened, processed foods, red meats, and—except for young children—whole milk and dairy products.

Good nutrition requires planning. This need not be a time-consuming or unpleasant chore. Rather than counting calories and nutrient values, we suggest using a modified form of the basic-food-group plan as your guide. The four basic groups are: dairy products; meats, eggs, fish, and poultry; fruits and vegetables; and breads and cereals. These are familiar to many of us from grade school.

There are a few problems with the food-group method of assessing eating patterns. It is possible to follow the plan and still have too much fat, salt, sugar, or cholesterol. However, within each group, food choices can be made according to the guidelines outlined above. Dairy products, for example, besides being limited, can be low-fat. We have added nuts and legumes to the meat group as protein sources low in saturated fats and cholesterol. Eggs, high in cholesterol, can be restricted.

We have also added to our charts categories of fats, water, and junk foods. Although anyone who eats meats and other animal products gets a sufficient amount of fat, we have added fats as a separate category to increase your awareness of how much much *extra* fat—especially unsaturated—you eat. Include here use of fat such as butter, margarine, mayonnaise, oil, even salad dressing with oil. You might be surprised at how much unnecessary fat you consume!

Many of us fail to drink enough water, so we've included this category. A good diet includes six to eight glasses of water each day.

Junk foods are those foods that supply calories without nutritional value—empty calories. Examples include candy, cake, and soft drinks.

Like so many aspects of our lives today, our diet is influenced by the age of technology. We no longer prepare all our foods at home. We use highly processed foods which have many of their natural nutrients removed; sometimes these are replaced or others are added. Often, foods are made with nonnutrient chemicals for flavor, color, or preservation. Foods are mixed so that many dishes contain a number of food groups. How, for example, to classify a cereal to which lots of sugar has been added? Is it a junk food or a bread and cereal food?

Food must therefore be selected wisely and carefully within each group. The chart on pages 106 and 107 lists some suggestions for nutritious food choices and food preparation. The readings listed at the end of this introduction provide additional guidance in making healthful selections. In *Nutrition Scoreboard,* Michael Jacobson outlines a way to "score" individual food products. He gives points for protein, naturally occurring carbohydrates, vitamins, minerals, and unsaturated fats. He subtracts points for sugar (and corn syrup), saturated fat, and high fat content.

We suggest learning to read food labels. Look for "polyunsaturated" fats, for example. The ingredients of many products are now listed, as are the nutrients provided in the food. When ingredients are given, they are listed in order of the amount contained in the food. The main ingredient appears first. Look for the following food additives and try to avoid them: nitrates or nitrites, caffeine, artificial sweeteners such as saccharin and cyclamates, and artificial flavors and colors. The preservatives BHA and BHT have not yet been found to be harmful but are certainly not necessary. Be wary, however; labels can be misleading. "Natural," for example, does not mean healthy. Sugar and honey are "natural" foods but are certainly not good for us.

Unfortunately, it is difficult to give complete guidelines for reading food labels. Few regulations exist for the standardization of labeling. There is no standard meaning to the word "organic," for example. In addition, so many substances are used in food preparation that it is not possible to note them all. It would be even more difficult to provide definitions.

The nutrition chart on page 105 gives the recommended daily intake of each food group by number of servings per day for adult females, males, children, adolescents, and pregnant and breast-feeding women. We have also provided an information chart on pages 106 and 107 which lists food groups, nutrient values, and examples of serving sizes and food choices. Tips on healthy ways to prepare foods are given.

We realize that food habits are often deeply ingrained. Food has different meanings for each of us, including protection, safety, and love. Food preparation connects us with our childhood and our cultural heritage. What we eat, how we eat, and when we eat are important to our individual identities. But we can learn to recognize harmful food habits and to overcome them.

In our society, eating is strongly influenced by business and advertising. The media inundate us with graphic displays of fattening, empty-calorie foods. Even supermarkets work against us—junk foods are temptingly placed on eye-level shelves, at checkout counters, and in the front of stores. It is unfortunate that sufficient public pressure has not been exerted to cause food manufacturers and distributors to advertise healthy products rather than junk food or to reduce the salt and sugar content of processed foods. Such pressure can be effective. Many baby foods are no longer made with salt or sugar because of public demand.

Changing eating attitudes and practices is possible, though it requires desire and commitment. The charts provided on pages 108 and 109 are samples of the kind of charts all family members can use to analyze their normal eating patterns. To determine whether your diet provides adequate nutrition, start by keeping a one-week record of your food intake. Choose a week during which your intake is representative of your general eating habits. Write down *everything* you eat and drink on a chart like the one provided. At the end of each day, decide in which food group or groups each item belongs. Use the facing page to analyze your intake according to your required food groups. Use the chart on page 109 to fill in the number of needed servings. To correct deficiencies and excesses, use the same type of chart to plan a week of healthful eating. Then, keep a diet history for at least one additional week. Check to see how well you've kept to your plan. If such written records help you maintain a sound diet, continue keeping them. You can use a small notebook or pad and follow the format given here. It is especially useful to maintain these records during pregnancy and breast-feeding, times during which good nutrition is especially vital.

Since eating is generally a family activity, we recommend meal planning as a family activity. Children need the same nutrients as do adults, although the needed amount differs and varies with age. Children often get as much of their required calories from snacks as from meals. Planning can make these nutritious as well. A good source for information about nutrition during childhood is *Growing Up Healthy: A Parent's Guide to Good Nutrition* by Myron Winick, M.D. (William Morrow and Company, Inc., New York, 1982).

As a science, nutrition is relatively new. It is not a required subject in all medical schools. Much is still unknown about our nutritional needs and how nutrients interact within our bodies. Controversies abound among nutrition experts. One area of great dispute is the question of vitamins. The National Academy of Sciences prepares RDAs—Recommended Dietary Allowances—for each vitamin, yet many nutritionists believe that these are far below our needs. Some proponents recommend routine use of vitamin supplements. Others feel that food is a better source of vitamins and minerals than pills. Yet there remains the question of how many vitamins and minerals we actually get in our diets of highly processed foods.

This introduction has focused on the problems associated with the typical American diet. These problems can lead to malnutrition created by overeating. It would be a grave oversight not to mention the other side of the nutrition problem—undernutrition. In most of the world and, indeed, among far too many people within our own country, undernutrition is a more common cause of suffering. Each year, *millions* of human beings die from protein or protein/calorie malnutrition—that is, starvation. Many of the affected are babies and young children. It is a sad and telling commentary on the world situation that here many of us suffer disease from overabundance while hunger is still very much a part of the human condition.

The following are good sources on nutrition: *Nutrition Scoreboard* by Michael Jacobson (Avon Books, New York, 1974) is available from the Center for Science in the Public Interest, 1755 S Street N.W., Washington, D.C. 20009. The center also publishes an excellent magazine, *Nutrition Action*. Write to them for information on subscribing. *Diet for a*

Small Planet by Frances Moore Lappé (Ballantine Books, New York, 1971) is must reading for vegetarians or anyone wanting to cut down on meat consumption. *Jane Brody's Nutrition Book* by Jane Brody (W. W. Norton and Co., New York, 1981) is rather expensive ($17.95) but an excellent overall nutritional guide. Perhaps it will be available in paperback by the time this book is published. The 1977 Senate Report on Nutrition, *Dietary Goals for the United States, 2nd Edition,* can be ordered from the U.S. Government Printing Office, Washington, D.C. 20402. The Surgeon General's nutritional report is included in the 1979 publication *Healthy People.* This also can be ordered from the U.S. Government Printing Office.

For more information on good eating during pregnancy and breast-feeding, we recommend *Nutrition for the Childbearing Year* by Jacqueline Gibson Gazella (Woodland Publishing Co., Inc., 230 Manitoba, Wayzata, Minnesota, 55301), available from the publisher, and *What Every Pregnant Woman Should Know: The Truth About Diet and Drugs in Pregnancy* by Gail Sforza Brewer (Penguin Books, New York, 1977).

For a discussion of the world food problem, we recommend reading *Food First: Beyond the Myth of Scarcity* by Frances Moore Lappé and Joseph Collins with Cary Fowler (Ballantine, 1979), available from the Institute for Food and Development Policy, 2588 Mission Street, San Francisco, California 94110.

Many other nutrition books are available. Some present controversial viewpoints. The more you read, the more information you will have with which to come to your own conclusions and make your own choices about healthful eating. We all must eat; why not eat well?

NUMBER OF DAILY REQUIRED FOOD GROUP SERVINGS FOR VARIOUS INDIVIDUALS

FOOD GROUP	ADULT FEMALE	ADULT MALE	CHILD	ADOLESCENT	PREGNANT WOMAN	BREAST-FEEDING WOMAN
DAIRY PRODUCTS	2	2	3-4; for weight loss: 3	at least 4	4	5
MEAT GROUP Meat Fish Eggs Poultry Beans Nuts Seeds	at least 2	at least 3	at least 2	at least 2	4	4-5
FRUITS AND VEGETABLES	at least 4-5; include: 1 citrus 1 leafy 1 yellow 3x/week	at least 4-6	at least 4-5	at least 4-5	at least 4-5	at least 4-5
BREADS AND CEREALS	at least 4; for weight loss: 2	at least 4-5; for weight loss: 3	at least 4-5; for weight loss: 3	at least 4-5	at least 4-5	at least 4-5
FATS	minimal					
WATER	at least 6-8 glasses					
JUNK FOODS	as few as possible; for weight loss: none				as few as possible	as few as possible

FACTS ABOUT THE FOOD GROUPS

FOOD GROUP	EXAMPLES OF ONE SERVING	MAJOR NUTRIENTS PROVIDED
DAIRY PRODUCTS	One 8-oz. glass milk 1 cup yogurt 1½ oz. hard cheese 1½ cups soft cheese (e.g., cottage cheese) 1½ cups ice cream	Protein Carbohydrates Vitamins: A, D, B_{12}, E Minerals: Calcium, phosphorus Almost everything except iron!

MEAT GROUP
  Meat
  Fish
  Eggs
  Poultry
  Beans (Legumes)
  Nuts
  Seeds
	1 egg
	3–4 oz. meat, fish, or
	  chicken
	3 oz. liver a week
	½ cup cooked beans
	  and rice
	2 tbsp. nut butter
		Protein, Vitamin B_{12}
		
		Iron, folic acid, B_{12}
		
		Protein, folic acid

FRUITS AND VEGETABLES	Citrus:
	1 orange, ½ grapefruit
	Green leafy:
	½ cup spinach, broc-
	  coli, greens
	Yellow:
	½ cantaloupe, 4 oz.
	  carrot
		Vitamin C
		
		Vitamin A
		Folic acid and iron
		Vitamin K
		Vitamin A
		
		All: Fiber

BREADS AND CEREALS	1 slice whole-grain
	  bread
	½ cup cooked rice
	1 small potato
	1 oz. cooked or dry
	  cereal
		Fiber
		Most of the Vitamin B complex
		Carbohydrates
		Whole-grain cereal—folic acid

FATS	2 teaspoons: oil (unsaturated is best) butter (saturated) mayonnaise (saturated) Found in animal products	Fats
WATER	1 8-oz. glass	Water
JUNK FOODS	cookies candy cake cookies doughnuts highly sweetened pro- cessed foods	None

WHAT THIS DOES IN YOUR BODY	COMMENTS SUGGESTIONS FOR COOKING AND PREPARING
Growth and healing Energy Healthy bones and teeth B_{12}—Healthy red blood cells	Except for young children, use low-fat or skimmed milk products. Powdered milk is low-fat and more economical; use in cooking if you can't drink. Ice cream provides nutrients, but also lots of fat and sugar. If you have lactose intolerance (get cramps and diarrhea from milk) use milk products such as yogurt and cheese.
Growth and healing To make good red blood cells	Limit eggs and red meats to avoid fats and cholesterol. Broiling or baking has less fat than frying. To make whole proteins mix: grains with: legumes, nuts, or milk seeds with: legumes or nuts for example: rice and beans, cereal and milk, peanut butter on whole-wheat
Prevents constipation and cancer of the intestine Vitamin C: aids healing; healthy gums Vitamin A: night vision; good skin Folic acid & iron: healthy red blood cells Vitamin K: blood clotting Calcium: healthy bones and teeth	Eat raw or steamed to get the most vitamins. Avoid overcooking. Reuse cooking water. The darker the green vegetable, the more iron it contains. Good for snacks.
Healthy nervous system Energy Healthy red blood cells	Avoid unnecessary processing such as mashing potatoes. Use potato skins for Vitamin C. Always use whole grains.
Help body use fat-soluble vitamins: A, D, E, K Protects organs and insulates body	Use mainly unsaturated fats—liquid at room temperature. An overly fatty diet has been implicated in heart disease and cancer.
The major chemical component of the body Necessary for all metabolic processes Necessary for healthy kidneys	
No value	Can fill you up with "empty calories" and prevent you from eating foods that contain nutrients. Lead to tooth decay. Lead to fat formation, implicated in arteriosclerosis, heart disease, and cancer. Implicated in behavioral disorders.

This chart was originally prepared by Margie Gold, M.D., and Ronnie Lichtman for childbirth classes at North Central Bronx Hospital. We thank Dr. Gold for allowing us to revise and reprint it.

WEEKLY DIET HISTORY/PLAN

MEAL	MONDAY	TUESDAY	WEDNES-DAY	THURS-DAY	FRIDAY	SATUR-DAY	SUNDAY
BREAK-FAST							
MID-MORN-ING SNACK(S)							
LUNCH							
MID-AFTER-NOON SNACK							
DINNER							
EVENING/NIGHT SNACKS							

FOOD GROUP ANALYSIS OF WEEKLY DIET

FOOD GROUP	FILL IN NUMBER OF SERV-INGS PER DAY*	MONDAY	TUESDAY	WEDNES-DAY	THURS-DAY	FRIDAY	SATUR-DAY	SUNDAY
DAIRY PRODUCTS								

MEAT GROUP
  Meat
  Fish
  Eggs
  Poultry
  Beans
  Nuts
  Seeds								

FRUITS AND VEGE-TABLES								
BREADS AND CEREALS								
FATS								
WATER								
JUNK FOODS								

* See "Number of Daily Required Food Group Servings for Various Individuals" (p. 105) to find appropriate number.

EXERCISE

Appreciation of the value of physical exercise dates back to ancient times. The early Greeks gave us the tradition of the Olympic games, and from the Romans we have the phrase "A sound mind in a sound body." Today, as physical labor is increasingly taken over by machines, we have had to develop a renewed awareness of the importance of exercise and to find alternative ways of incorporating it into our lives.

Exercise serves three distinct purposes. It can develop endurance through its effects on the heart and circulatory (cardiovascular) system. The exact effect of exercise on the circulatory system is not entirely understood. It is known, however, that it has both preventive and symptom-relieving functions in heart diseases such as angina pectoris—chest pain due to a decrease in the blood flow to the heart muscle.

Exercise also builds muscular strength and muscular flexibility. Muscle strength and flexibility increase the enjoyment of such activities as athletics and dance. They ease everyday tasks like stair climbing. An important benefit of flexibility is that it reduces the likelihood of injury from sports or other activities.

Exercise follows the principle of specificity. Various types of exercises must be practiced to achieve all three purposes. Strength training will not improve cardiovascular endurance. Exercises intended for flexibility will not develop strength or endurance. Endurance exercises include walking, swimming, bicycling, jogging, and running. Strength can be developed by training with weights. Flexibility is enhanced through stretches or yoga.

Gradualness is important when beginning an exercise program. It takes six to eight weeks for the effects of training to become apparent. All increases in activity should be made in small daily increments.

If you have been inactive, do not undertake sudden, intense exercise. Almost everyone can tolerate increased walking and that is a good starting point. If your health is not optimal, it is recommended that you consult your practitioner before attempting further exercise. Stress testing may be necessary. This involves monitoring heart function during controlled activity.

Every exercise period should begin with a warm-up. Warm-up should include stretching and conditioning—jogging over distance or in place. The amount of time needed for warm-up depends on the intensity and duration of your exercise session. Anywhere from five to thirty minutes may be required.

The intensity and duration of your exercises will depend on your physical condition and state of training. Intensity—the level at which you exercise—will increase as you train. Duration can be as short as fifteen to twenty minutes a day at first. This can be increased to as much as one or two hours a day, keeping in mind the principle of gradualness. The more tired you are when you exercise, the more prone you become to injury. Stop before reaching the point of fatigue.

In order for an exercise program to be beneficial, it must be followed at least two days per week. Three to five days per week is ideal for a training program.

One reassuring fact about exercising is that you will always note improvement. The older you are, however, the slower the change will be. Slow changes can be expected during pregnancy as well.

Good nutrition is essential for anyone who exercises. Nutritional deficiencies can predispose you to injury. Use the section "Nutrition" (p. 100) along with this section for best results.

To avoid injury, learn to listen to your own body. Sore joints, shortness of breath, and overall weariness are messages from your body. If at any time you wake up feeling unusually listless, unable to muster up the enthusiasm to perform your usual training program, it is wise to obey that feeling. Your own body is your best protector, provided you allow it to be.

Not surprisingly, the desire for physical fitness has been the basis for the creation of a lucrative market. Elaborate equipment, fashionable clothing, and memberships in luxurious health clubs sell at exorbitant prices. None of these are necessary for participation in beneficial activities. The reality of economics must always be considered in planning programs designed to optimize health.

In the charts that follow, we have provided a way for you to record the exercise you perform on a routine basis. For examples of specific exercises and directions for their performance, we recommend the following books:

Nutrition, Weight Control and Exercise, Frank I. Katch and William D. McArdle, Houghton Mifflin, Boston, 1977.
Condition Fundamentals, Edward C. Olson, Part of Merrill Sports Series, Charles E. Merrill Publishing Co., Ohio, 1968.
The Aerobics Way, Kenneth Cooper, Bantam Books, New York, 1977.
Many books on yoga and dance may be valuable as well.

The following books describe specific exercises to be done during pregnancy and the postpartum period. They also discuss the role and value of exercise during these times and provide guidelines for planning pregnancy and postpartum activity programs:

Essential Exercises for the Childbearing Year, Elizabeth Noble, Houghton Mifflin, Boston, 1976.

Moving Through Pregnancy, Elisabeth Bing, Bantam Books, New York, 1980.

The Exercise Plus Pregnancy Program, Lazar and Olinda Cedeno and Carole Monroe, William Morrow and Company, Inc., New York, 1980.

Further information on exercise is available from the American Heart Association National Center, 7320 Greenville Avenue, Dallas, Texas 75231, and The President's Council on Physical Fitness, Washington, D.C.

Since exercise can be a daily, lifelong pursuit, the charts in this section are samples only. The first chart shows you how you can record repetitions and sets accomplished at each exercise session. Each time you perform an exercise it is called a repetition. A set is a group of repetitions. Space is also provided for distance, time, and heart rate if you walk, jog, bicycle, run, or swim. Time and heart rate will help you monitor the intensity of cardiovascular exercises. Recording them will enable you to follow your own progress. The second chart shows a record of monthly changes in body measurements and weight for males and females that occur as you work out. Keeping track of these results will undoubtedly increase your motivation for continuing your program. If you wish to continue to chart your exercise progress, we suggest keeping further records in a small, inexpensive notebook that can be a companion to this book. Specific charts can also be kept for pregnancy and postpartum exercises, since the activities may be different.

The authors wish to acknowledge and thank Steven Lichtman, M.Ed., M.S., for his invaluable assistance in preparing this section. He provided the research and information on which the section was based and the charts developed.

EXERCISE RECORD

EXERCISE	DATE:																		
WALKING	Distance																		
	Time/Heart Rate																		
JOGGING RUNNING SWIMMING BICYCLING	Distance																		
	Time/Heart Rate																		
	Repetitions																		
	Sets																		
	Repetitions																		
	Sets																		
	Repetitions																		
	Sets																		
	Repetitions																		
	Sets																		
	Repetitions																		
	Sets																		
	Repetitions																		
	Sets																		
	Repetitions																		
	Sets																		
	Repetitions																		
	Sets																		
	Repetitions																		
	Sets																		
	Repetitions																		
	Sets																		
	Repetitions																		
	Sets																		

MONTHLY BODY MEASUREMENTS AND WEIGHT FOR ADULT FEMALE

DATE								
NECK								
CHEST								
WAIST/Abdomen								
RIGHT BICEPS (Upper Arm)								
LEFT BICEPS (Upper Arm)								
RIGHT FOREARM								
LEFT FOREARM								
HIPS								
RIGHT THIGH								
LEFT THIGH								
RIGHT CALF								
LEFT CALF								
WEIGHT								

MONTHLY BODY MEASUREMENTS AND WEIGHT FOR ADULT MALE

DATE								
NECK								
CHEST								
ABDOMEN								
RIGHT BICEPS (Upper Arm)								
LEFT BICEPS (Upper Arm)								
RIGHT FOREARM								
LEFT FOREARM								
RIGHT THIGH								
LEFT THIGH								
RIGHT CALF								
LEFT CALF								
WEIGHT								

Health Issues

Informed Consent

As the science of medicine probes deeper into the intricacies of biologic processes and increases its reliance on complex and technological methods of diagnosis and treatment, personal decision-making in health care seems ever more remote. Patients' records are programmed into computers, and sophisticated statistical probabilities are used to determine treatment choices; new drugs and machines are continually placed on the market. Surgeons operate with microscopes, and doctors change and manipulate our chemical balances. The patient is too often confused and feels unable to participate fully in his or her own care.

We believe the individual must maintain the right to decide what is to be done to and for his or her own body, regardless of the scientific complexity of the problem. The courts have generally upheld this right, except in the special circumstances of emergencies, or in the case of children or the mentally impaired. This means that health professionals have a responsibility to provide us with information about our bodies; we are entitled to know what tests are taken when we seek care, what the results are, what diseases and disorders we have, and what treatments are available. We have the right to know what the expected benefits of these treatments are, what the probability of their success is, what risks and what side effects exist. We have the right to be told about alternative treatments and what we can expect if we refuse to be treated. We must be given the opportunity to ask any and all questions and to refuse treatment. If any aspect of care is experimental, we must be so informed. All information must be clear and understandable. Together, these rights comprise *informed consent*.

The following chart is a guideline for situations in which you must give informed consent—if you are advised to take medication, to have surgery, radiation, or other special therapies. Use it to make sure that you are accorded the full right of informed consent.

In the case of your children, rights are less clear. Generally, parents have the right to consent to care for their children. A doctor or hospital may, however, go to court to request that the judge appoint a guardian legally empowered to consent to treatment when parents have refused. This is usually done for treatments considered lifesaving, such as a blood transfusion for a child whose parents have refused it for religious reasons.

For further discussion of informed consent and other rights of patients, see George Annas's excellent guide, *The Rights of Hospital Patients,* prepared as an American Civil Liberties Union publication (Avon Books, New York, 1975). We also refer you to the American Hospital Association's *A Patient's Bill of Rights* and to *A Pregnant Patient's Bill of Rights* (p. 180), distributed by the Committee on Patient's Rights.

CHART FOR INFORMED CONSENT

Description of Diagnostic Tests:
Explanation of Diagnosis:
Description of Treatment(s):
Expected Benefits:
Probability of Success:
Risks, Side Effects:
Alternative Treatment(s):
Expected Benefits of Alternative Treatment(s):
Probability of Success of Alternative Treatment(s):
Risks, Side Effects of Alternative Treatment(s):
Expected Outcome of No Treatment:
Experimental Aspects of Treatment(s):

A PATIENT'S BILL OF RIGHTS

1. The patient has the right to considerate and respectful care.
2. The patient has the right to obtain from his physician complete current information concerning his diagnosis, treatment, and prognosis in terms the patient can be reasonably expected to understand. When it is not medically advisable to give such information to the patient, the information should be made available to an appropriate person in his behalf. He has the right to know, by name, the physician responsible for coordinating his care.
3. The patient has the right to receive from his physician information necessary to give informed consent prior to the start of any procedure and/or treatment. Except in emergencies, such information for informed consent should include but not necessarily be limited to the specific procedure and/or treatment, the medically significant risks involved, and the probable duration of incapacitation. Where medically significant alternatives for care or treatment exist, or when the patient requests information concerning medical alternatives, the patient has the right to such information. The patient also has the right to know the name of the person responsible for the procedures and/or treatment.
4. The patient has the right to refuse treatment to the extent permitted by law and to be informed of the medical consequences of his action.
5. The patient has the right to every consideration of his privacy concerning his own medical care program. Case discussion, consultation, examination, and treatment are confidential and should be conducted discreetly. Those not directly involved in his care must have the permission of the patient to be present.
6. The patient has the right to expect that all communications and records pertaining to his care should be treated as confidential.
7. The patient has the right to expect that within its capacity a hospital must make reasonable response to the request of a patient for services. The hospital must provide evaluation, service, and/or referral as indicated by the urgency of the case. When medically permissible, a patient must be transferred to another facility only after he has received complete information and explanation concerning the needs for and alternatives to such a transfer. The institution to which the patient is to be transferred must first have accepted the patient for transfer.
8. The patient has the right to obtain information as to any relationship of his hospital to other health care and educational institutions insofar as his care is concerned. The patient has the right to obtain information as to the existence of any professional relationships among individuals, by name, who are treating him.
9. The patient has the right to be advised if the hospital proposes to engage in or perform human experimentation affecting his care or treatment. The patient has the right to refuse to participate in such research projects.
10. The patient has the right to expect reasonable continuity of care. He has the right to know in advance what appointment times and physicians are available and where. The patient has the right to expect that the hospital will provide a mechanism whereby he is informed by his physician or a delegate of the physician of the patient's continuing health care requirements following discharge.
11. The patient has the right to examine and receive an explanation of his bill regardless of source of payment.
12. The patient has the right to know what hospital rules and regulations apply to his conduct as a patient.

Reprinted with permission of the American Hospital Association, copyright © 1975.

Discussing the "Unspeakable": Some Social Factors and Their Relation to Health

Some of the most critical health problems that afflict individuals and families are things many people find difficult to discuss with practitioners. Though record-keeping might be helpful, it often seems out of the question. Rape and domestic violence, for example, are seen as social problems but can cause devastating mental and physical health problems. Antihomosexual prejudice can make it hard for gay people to get adequate medical treatment. Alcoholism and other substance abuse may be seen as too embarrassing or threatening to bring into the open. Some of these subjects are sensitive because of sexism or public ignorance; it should not be embarrassing to be a victim of assault or of a disease such as alcoholism.

In this chapter, we will offer some guidelines for seeking treatment and support for these "unspeakable" problems. We will also deal with some of the main health issues raised and their possible long-term effects. Where it is indicated, we will show how record-keeping can be organized and why it is useful. At the end of each topic, you will find suggestions for locating help.

One great advance for the health movement during the last two decades was the emergence "out of the closet" of open discussion of many subjects. The demands by gays for dignity and equal rights, the movement for reform in the treatment of rape victims, and in the last few years the emergence of literature and support groups for incest victims are all positive examples of this trend. But medical schools and other professional training institutions are still not teaching practitioners to detect or handle many of these problems. Health-care providers who have been through special classes on detecting batterment or child abuse, for example, are amazed to discover how many cases "suddenly" turn up in their practice. Yet these better educated practitioners are still too few and far between. Often, it is not possible to locate someone who is both sympathetic and highly trained.

We believe it is important for people to learn to find help within the system of care that exists, to learn to cope with the inadequacies of that system and make sure their needs are met. This is vitally necessary on an individual level and can often be the key to actual survival. Socially it is also necessary to help educate practitioners to the reality of the world around them. These guidelines may help you in obtaining care:

Seek Self-help and Support Groups

These are excellent sources for referral to sympathetic practitioners. They also provide the extremely valuable help of those who have "been there" before you. Because they work in a specialized area, they may have knowledge that is not available to most practitioners. The whole range of peer-support organizations, from Alcoholics Anonymous to rape and incest victim discussion groups, have in common an ability to help people cope with problems and rebuild their lives. You may also find strength in the act of reaching out to help others.

Be Bold and Speak Up

Make sure that you get the help you need. Don't let a physical or mental health problem get out of hand because of embarrassment. If you need support, take someone with you if possible—but go.

The Practitioner Must Earn Your Trust

Remember that though the situation has improved somewhat, many practitioners are still unprepared to deal with difficult subjects. You need the professional assistance they provide, but it is wise to remember that they may well share the same hangups and limitations as the rest of society. You may find you are not being taken seriously, as in the case of a woman who is advised to stop provoking the husband who beats her. Change practitioners if necessary, and reserve your emotional trust until you see that you are being taken seriously, being dealt with as a person, and receiving the help for which you came.

In the following pages, we will discuss some of the specific health hazards associated with "unspeakable" or sensitive subjects and list referral and self-help agencies for each.

ALCOHOLISM AND DRUG ABUSE

Alcoholism is a deadly disease. It is a contributing factor in countless other health problems. The alcoholic is more likely to develop high blood pressure, diabetes, gastritis, anxiety, depression, and sexual problems (including impotence). Alcoholics and drug abusers become accident prone. Half the fatal car accidents in the country involve alcohol. Deterioration of family life occurs, sometimes bringing direct physical danger to other family members, including violence such as wife-beating and child abuse.

Denial, the refusal to admit or discuss an alcohol or drug problem, stands between the addict and treatment. Because of this denial, it is difficult to offer simple solutions or suggestions for help. Drug addiction and overuse can be given a cloak of respectability when they involve drugs legally obtained with a doctor's prescription. Some alcoholics argue that they "only drink beer"—though alcohol in any form is the same drug. Others rationalize that they are not breaking any law. There are several standardized tests available for self-diagnosis. You can request copies of these from your local chapter of the National Council on Alcoholism or Alcoholics Anonymous.

Each alcoholic has been estimated to harmfully affect an average of four other persons in his family and more than sixteen friends and business associates in the community. The families of alcoholics and drug abusers are subjected to many difficulties. It seems impossible to help the addict; it may begin to seem impossible for the family to help themselves. Support organizations exist for these families, and counseling that is available through mental-health clinics can help family members withstand stress and cope together.

Sometimes people let a sense of embarrassment or shame keep them away from help for a drug or alcohol problem. They may believe they are protecting themselves or their position in the community. In fact, this is simply another excuse to avoid facing the extent of their problem. Those who have joined support groups or entered treatment centers for their addiction have found out how universal the problem can be, afflicting professionals and homemakers, politicians and blue-collar workers. In all alcoholism and drug-abuse treatment, great emphasis is placed on confidentiality.

To find medical help for alcoholism, call your local office of the National Council on Alcoholism. For alcohol and other drug abuse, medical help can also be located through one of the treatment facilities in your area, including hospital detoxification centers and halfway houses.

A partial list of support organizations follows. With each, you should look for a local chapter listed in your telephone book. If you have difficulty locating a chapter in your area, call one of the treatment facilities or look up another of the listed support organizations and seek suggestions from them.

> Alcoholics Anonymous
> Al-Anon (for families of alcoholics)
> Al-Ateen (for teenage relatives of alcoholics)
> Narcotics Anonymous
> Recovery, Inc.

BATTERMENT (WIFE-BEATING)

Batterment may affect up to one third of the families in the United States. Battering is a crime even when it occurs between married people. It causes a large number of mental and physical health problems. It may result in the death of *either* person. Often it goes on to include child abuse. The batterer often promises to stop, but to find a solution requires separation or long-term counseling.

Although battering may appear at any time in a relationship, there are certain times when it is most likely to begin: immediately after marriage, during the first pregnancy, upon retirement, or with the onset of senility. Probably the most common onset is during pregnancy. Many reasons have been proposed for this, including jealousy of the fetus and stress on the whole family. It can pose grave dangers to the unborn child as well as to the mother-to-be. Besides the dangers of direct injury, the ongoing stress and fear can give rise to complications in pregnancy.

Battering can be terribly difficult for a woman to discuss with her practitioner. She may have trouble admitting it to herself. The woman may fear the most hostile response: "What did you do to provoke him?" or "You must deserve it." She may shrink from opening up the most painful intimacies of her marriage or fear further abuse if her husband discovers she has spoken out. Sometimes a battered woman believes that reaching for help will be the beginning of the end of the relationship. This may be true, since the batterer often resists change and forces a choice between more abuse and a complete break.

This avoidance of honesty with oneself, friends, and practitioners is a danger to the battered woman. The chart on page 124, "Recognizing the Developing Pattern of Abuse," is designed both to help recognize the abusive trend and to provide a partial record. Dr. Lenore Walker, in her book *The Battered Woman,* describes a three-stage cycle which is helpful in understanding wife abuse.

Phase 1: the tension-building stage. This includes minor battering incidents, isolated temper outbursts. Gradually, tension increases. Some couples can keep this phase going for long periods of time with very gradual intensification. The incidence of these minor episodes grows more frequent; it becomes less possible to keep the tension in check.

Phase 2: the acute battering incident. The batterer's rage is out of control. It may be triggered by an external event or by the man's internal state. This stage is brief, lasting no more than two to twenty-four hours. This is the time when the police are most likely to be called.

Phase 3: contrition, apology, and kind, loving behavior. The batterer knows he has gone too far and tries to make up. The tension is gone, and a period of calm follows. The batterer is sorry, loving, even charming. He swears he will improve himself—for example, by giving up drinking. This period has no distinct end. It blends gradually into the reemergence of small incidents and a recurrence of Phase 1.

As in the section "Long-term Illness," it is not really possible to provide the necessary charts for documentation in this workbook. There is also the danger that the discovery of records or documentation might provoke further abuse. There are solutions to this problem.

The chart on page 125, "Documenting Abuse," shows the information that a battered woman needs to report. We suggest copying this chart into a notebook which can be hidden around the house or even outside the house, with friends or family, or at a place of employment. The same should be done with the chart "Recognizing the Developing Pattern of Abuse." While it is not always possible to fill in every category for documentation, the more information the better. It can help you in seeking counseling and in establishing a sound legal position in states that consider fault in separation or divorce. If charges of assault or battery must be made, documentation provides backup evidence. There is also a psychological advantage to record-keeping, as the woman begins to be honest with herself about her situation and can take steps to improve it.

Most battering involves a series of incidents growing more severe. Even if you think an incident will not happen again, you should record it. If you find you are already in a cycle of battering, go back and record as much information as you have on earlier incidents. This documentation is extremely valuable when seeking counseling or legal action, such as separation, divorce, or protective court orders. If you are afraid this record will be found by the batterer, you can think of a place to hide it where he does not look. Possibly a friend will keep your records at her house, or you can keep them at your office or job.

In many cities, battered women's shelters or crisis lines exist. If you cannot locate one, you may find help through a rape crisis line, women's switchboard, YWCA switchboard, or through a mental-health crisis line. Child-protection services may also be a resource as battering often goes on to affect children physically and certainly does severe psychological harm.

For more information, we recommend reading:

The Battered Woman by Lenore Walker (Harper & Row, 1979); *Stopping Wife Abuse* by Jennifer Baker (Anchor Press/Doubleday, 1979); and *Conjugal Crime* by Terry Davidson (Hawthorn Books, 1978). *Conjugal Crime* contains a directory of shelters and crisis lines.

RECOGNIZING THE DEVELOPING PATTERN OF ABUSE

ABUSIVE BEHAVIOR	WHAT (IF ANYTHING) TRIGGERED INCIDENT —CIRCUMSTANCES	LIST *ALL* DATES AND TIMES WHEN ABUSE OCCURRED
Shouting		
Name calling and verbal abuse		
Verbal threats		
Physical threats (waving fists, etc.)		
Violence against objects (breaking windows, furniture, etc.)		
Violence against others (including pets, etc.)		
Violence against spouse choking		
pushing		
slapping		
punching		
kicking		
biting		
other (specify)_______		
Use of weapons knife		
gun		
piece of furniture		
shoe		
club/blunt instrument		
other (specify)		
Other abuse (specify)_______		

DOCUMENTING ABUSE
Use this outline to make a full record of each incident.

Date:

Time:

Abusive behavior:

Location and appearance of room:

Witnesses:

Circumstances (what triggered abuse):

Quotes (what was said):

Drugs or alcohol used by batterer:

Pictures taken of your injuries or the room:

Medical help:

   Doctor or hospital name and address:

   Date of visit:

   Injuries:

   Treatment or care received:

Police:

   Time police arrived:

   Badge numbers of police officers:

   Actions taken by police:

Notes and comments, including damage to clothes and property:

CHILD ABUSE—INCLUDING SEXUAL ABUSE

Child abuse includes battering, neglect, and sexual abuse. Sexual abuse of children takes the forms of rape, incest, and other types of molestation; it is most often committed by a trusted adult, either an acquaintance or a family member. Although battering may be easier to detect than sexual abuse, since it leaves obvious evidence in the form of scars, burns, and broken bones, sexual abuse of children can leave recognizable, if less clearcut, symptoms.

Sexual exploitation, especially incest, is far more common than is generally suspected. It is extremely difficult for victims to discuss, even long after they are grown and removed from the exploitative situation. The stigma of shame and fear is great. There have been cases of adults who were in therapy for years for other problems before they could admit a childhood experience of incest.

Abuse must be stopped and the child must be protected. If the child finds treatment quickly, a good recovery may be made. But where incest or other sexual abuse is not discovered and stopped, and the family is not treated, the experience can leave lifelong scars. Suicide rates among incest victims are high, as are mental illness, alcoholism, and drug abuse.

The problem of child abuse is different from others discussed in this chapter, since it is generally impossible for the victim to seek care and extremely rare for the abusing adult to do so. For this reason, self-help groups cannot be considered a primary resource although they do exist to help parents who are trying to cope and change. They do not meet the needs of the whole family. Also, the idea of confidentiality with or "reserving your trust" in practitioners does not apply in the same way as it does for situations involving adults.

It is up to the many adults who touch on the lives of abused children to recognize the problem and take action. It can save the child's life or prevent tragic consequences. A list of symptoms often exhibited by abused children is given in the section "Some Symptoms of Abuse" (p. 129). Inability to "read" symptoms of abuse can keep some people from intervening as can denial (disbelief that such a thing could actually be happening), and uncertainty as to what action should be taken. The long-cherished notion in our society that "a man's home is his castle" protects abusive adults, both men and women. Many people are reluctant to involve themselves in what they see as somebody else's family affairs.

Child abuse is an emergency. If you know or suspect a child is being abused, your first responsibility is to protect that child. Some experts and individuals seek to keep the family together as much as possible in treatment, but this goal must never take precedence over protecting the victim. By intervening, you can help stop the violence which is taught from generation to generation. Battering parents were often battered children themselves, and incest victims often go on to molest their own children or to marry molesters. These patterns of family relationships are learned at such an early age that they often operate on a subconscious level, creating parents who cannot break the cycle without help.

You cannot rely on others to intervene for you. Reporting laws have now been enacted in every state. These laws protect you from lawsuits if your report is made in good faith. Almost all states provide confidentiality for the person making the report. Most such laws also require certain professionals such as doctors, teachers, and counselors to report any suspicions of abuse. Some carry stiff penalties for failure to report. However, even in those states with the strictest laws, underreporting is still a tremendous problem.

Child protection services have improved dramatically in the past several years. Sometimes professionals fail to report because they fear the weaknesses in the system of care available to abused children, such as the inadequacy of foster homes. Exposure is more likely to be helpful than harmful. It may be painful, for example, for a child to retell the story of abuse several times, but it is far less damaging than the continuation of the abuse in secret.

Another excuse for failure to report is the belief that as long as some action is being taken, such as one member of the family receiving treatment, the situation is improving. This denies the entire family access to badly needed services. Child-protection agencies are able to use many resources for treatment: pediatricians and other medical specialists, law enforcement officers, psychologists and mental health counselors, social workers, judges and the entire judicial system.

There are many ways you may find out about child abuse. If a child tells you, *believe the child.* A child's report of abuse, no matter how incredible to you, must be considered evidence of abuse and reported to a child-protection agency. After all, both battering and sexual abuse can go on "in the best families." They occur across all social and ethnic lines. It is possible for someone who is considered a pillar of the community to be a child abuser as well. If you try to investigate on your own, you may encounter denial by the abusing adult and can even put the child in greater danger.

Sometimes you will learn of abuse because the child is a member of your family, and you or other family members have witnessed abusive behavior. Venereal disease in a child is another indicator of abuse. If you are a teacher, you may notice a student who is continually bruised and injured. Any such evidence should be reported to a child-protection service.

However, it may be that you have no hard evidence. You may believe or sense that something is wrong, but feel your suspicions are vague and there are other possible explanations. Unfortunately, asking the adult does not provide reliable information, because a negative answer cannot necessarily be believed. A direct question to the child might not bring a truthful answer either. The child's trust in adults has been broken. It is likely, especially with sexual abuse, that threats will have been made to enforce the child's silence.

One positive step you can take is to open communication with the child. Often adult reluctance to discuss sex with children and refusal to believe the possibility of sexual molestation leave children surrounded by a wall of silence. Your openness can show that you are one adult who is not afraid to discuss the problem. You might start by discussing good and bad kinds of touch, and how sometimes people try to touch you in a bad way. You can assure them that they do not need to obey someone just because he or she is a grown-up, and they should not keep physical approaches secret. You can also talk about their right to control their own bodies, and how we all have the right to do only those things that are comfortable to us physically—we should not be pushed into touch or other behavior that feels wrong or is frightening. Directly and indirectly, you will be telling the child whose side you are on. This is vitally important information.

Again, *believe the child!* No matter how difficult it seems to believe, or how information about abuse is put forward. Children cannot fantasize about things they have not been exposed to. This is particularly true for sexuality: Children simply do not conjure up imaginary accounts of sexual activity. The child has witnessed something, and direct experience is the most likely source.

How can you protect your child, and what social measures can help improve the situation for all children? More programs are needed that provide support to families in crisis. Parent-aid programs assist abusive parents by providing a counselor—another parent—who can help them learn to manage pressure without harming the children. Prediction programs try to pinpoint families that are at high risk of child abuse and provide parenting education and other intervention before abuse takes place. These programs need to be supported and expanded.

The greatest single step to prevent sexual abuse and/or detect it early would be a universal program of sex education in the schools, beginning in the very youngest grades. Going beyond "the birds and the bees," children should be taught about good and bad touch, and where they can turn for help if something happens which frightens or harms them.

Within your family, your children should hear these same messages. You can respect their need for security and their reluctance to do things that make them uncomfortable, whether these things are social or physical. Parents sometimes push children to be physically affectionate, even with people who make those same parents uncomfortable. Children should not be forced to be affectionate, or taught to confuse kissing a relative with respect for older family members.

Let your children know they are free to talk to you. This means remaining open to what the child says, not becoming angry when his or her opinion differs from yours. It does not mean never showing anger to your child, which would be unhealthy and is an impossible goal. Teach children they can trust you with the truth, and then believe them when they speak. This protects them from being victims of abuse, and it also lays a sound foundation for family relationships.

Pamphlets and additional information are available from: National Committee for Prevention of Child Abuse, Publishing Dept., 332 S. Michigan Ave., Suite 1250, Chicago, Ill. 60604, (312) 663-3520; American Humane Society–Children's Division, 9725 E. Hampton, Denver, Col. 80231, (303) 695-0811.

We recommend reading:

Kiss Daddy Goodnight, Louise Armstrong, Hawthorne Books, 1978.
Father's Days, Katherine Brady, Seaview Books, 1979.
Conspiracy of Silence, Sandra Butler, New Glide Publications, 1978.

Betrayal of Innocence: Incest and Its Devastation, Susan Forward, Penguin Books, 1978.
The Battered Child, edited by C. Henry Kempe and Ray E. Helfer, 3rd Ed., University of Chicago Press, 1980.
Physical and Sexual Abuse of Children: Causes and Treatment, David Walters, Indiana University Press, 1975.

Some Symptoms of Abuse

DIRECT EVIDENCE OF ABUSE

A child's report of abuse
Venereal disease
Battered appearance, including bruises, burns, broken bones

POSSIBLE EVIDENCE OF ABUSE

(No one symptom is conclusive, but a few or more indicate a troubled child who needs help and may be a victim of abuse.)

Vaginal discharge or bleeding
Discharge from the penis
Sudden changes in behavior:
    sleeping habits
    developing a fear of the dark
    avoidance or fear of a certain person
    eating habits
    talkative child who becomes quiet
    school habits and grades
Mysterious appearance of toys or money
Withdrawal from friends and playmates
Avoidance of physical activity such as gym class
Fear of undressing in front of others, as in locker room
Development of general physical ailments:
    stomachaches
    headaches
    gastrointestinal problems
Vague references to trouble at home
Dramatic change in appearance, suddenly sloppy or very neat
Taking a great number of baths

In a young child, regressing to an earlier stage:
    thumb sucking
    whining
    clinging
In a teenager, development of self-destructive behavior:
    drug abuse
    alcoholism
    promiscuity
    prostitution

Masturbation and sexual curiosity: These are difficult to evaluate, because standards of normal behavior vary greatly in different families and cultures. We consider masturbation, curiosity about the human body, and investigation such as "playing doctor" to be activities often found in normal, healthy children. However, if the child seems anxious or obsessed, it may be a sign of trouble. Explicitly sexual play or urgent curiosity about the genitals of people or animals may be symptoms of a child who is being sexually abused.

RAPE

Rape is a crime of violence. Any woman may become a rape victim. Victims have included baby girls, expectant mothers, nuns, and women in their eighties. Rape may take place outside on the street or in a car, or it may happen inside your home or near your job. The rapist may be a complete stranger, an acquaintance, a casual friend, or even a family member.

Rape gives rise to a number of physical and mental health problems. The section "What Treatment Should Include" on page 131 lists medical and legal steps the rape victim can expect. Because prosecuting the rapist makes further demands on the victim's emotional resources and abilities, we have also included a chart "Documenting the Rape—What the Victim Needs to Remember" on page 132.

Bruises and other physical injuries, emotional shock, and the danger of venereal disease and pregnancy are the immediate consequences of rape. Long-term aftereffects can include insomnia, depression, and the development of extreme fears (phobias). These may include fear of crowds, fear of being outdoors, fear of being alone, and sexual fears. Sexual problems may include vaginismus (constriction making intercourse painful or impossible), loss of the ability to have an orgasm, and a loss of vaginal lubrication or genital sensation. Marital problems sometimes develop in families that have difficulty communicating about the rape. If any of these symptoms occur, be sure that your practitioner or counselor knows about the rape and can assist you in finding a solution.

Rape was one of the first social/health issues to draw the focus of the women's liberation movement in the late 1960s and early 1970s. The traditional mentality that blamed the victim was sharply disputed. Treatment methods of police and hospitals were targets of militant demands for greater sensitivity and better care. The need for support and counseling was stressed, and rape crisis lines developed around the country. The sense of shame and helplessness some rape victims experienced was addressed, with "Speak-Outs" on rape where victims discussed the problem publicly. Treatment of rape victims has come a long way in the past ten years. Unfortunately, it still has a long way to go. Use the chart "What Treatment Should Include" to be sure you get the help you need.

After you have received medical care and made a police report, you must readjust to your life and overcome the emotional aftereffects of rape. Often, quite a long time may pass before you must go to court to testify against the rapist. The passage of time and a desire to forget may result in the memory of the actual events of the rape becoming hazy. We suggest you use the chart "Documenting the Rape—What the

Victim Needs to Remember" (p. 132) to write a report you can refer to for legal needs at a later date.

We strongly recommend that rape victims contact their local rape crisis line for assistance and counseling. You will find valuable advice and support there. You may wish to participate in group discussions with fellow victims. Support from others in your situation helps you understand your own reactions and often helps speed recovery from the trauma.

For more information, we recommend reading:

> *Sexual Assault: Confronting Rape in America,* Nancy Gager and Cathleen Schurr, Grosset & Dunlap, 1976.
>
> *Rape: Victims of Crisis,* Ann Wolbert Burgess and Lynda Lytle Holmstrom, Robert J. Brady Co., 1974. This book is oriented toward counselors and other professionals but has useful information for the average reader.
>
> *Men Who Rape: The Psychology of the Offender,* A. Nicholas Groth with H. Jean Birnbaum, Plenum Press, 1979. Many rape victims express a need to understand the rapist and the reasons for rape; this book focuses on the rapist.

What Treatment Should Include

THE POLICE SHOULD

> Take a written statement and have you sign it.
> Show you mug shots, if the rapist is a stranger and has not been arrested.
> Collect evidence at the scene of the crime (such as bed sheets, your clothes, etc.).
> Make sure that you have a medical examination.

THE MEDICAL EXAMINATION WILL INCLUDE

Tests for Legal Evidence

These tests all help in identification. They do not prove rape. Negative findings on these tests do not disprove rape—in fact, they may support your account of the rape.

> Pelvic examination—taking smears for presence of sperm and similar fluids.
> Combing of pubic hairs—to find loose hairs of the rapist's. A few of your own hairs will be pulled for comparison with loose hairs.
> Saliva test—swabbing the mouth for traces of saliva to help in identification or traces of sperm if oral sex was part of the rape.
> Swabbing the rectum—if anal rape was performed.
> Scraping under fingernails—for traces of the rapist's skin or hair.

If you have visible physical injuries, photographs should be taken. The doctor may note them on the report.

Treatment

Treatment for injuries.

Antibiotics. You should be offered the choice of having penicillin to treat possible venereal disease or of waiting (if you prefer) to see if disease develops and treatment is necessary. Some hospitals do tests for venereal disease as part of the exam, but the reliability of these tests is questionable so soon after the rape.

"Morning-after Shot." You should be offered the choice of having this preventive measure against pregnancy, which is a very high dose of hormones including estrogen (DES). You may wish to wait and find out if you are pregnant rather than taking the shot. It does have side effects, including nausea and some cramping. It is also thought to be a possible cancer-causing agent both for the woman and for the infant if the shot does not work and a pregnancy continues.

Documenting the Rape—What the Victim Needs to Remember

Use these questions to write your own report:

Date, time, and location of the rape:

Description of the rapist or rapists. How many were there?

Other people involved: Other victims

                    Witnesses

                    Accomplices of the rapist

What led up to the rape:

Account of the rape itself:
  Acts the rapist performed:
  Acts he forced you to perform:
  What he said:
  What type of threats were made:
  What type of force was used:
  What type of weapons (if any) were used:

Injuries:

Injuries visible after the rape:

Other injuries (Bruises and other injuries may show up later, in 1–3 days. Document these by showing them to someone, preferably a health practitioner or police officer. Marks will have faded again by the time you go to court.):

What you did after the rape:

3.

Reproductive Health

Menstrual History

Many women associate keeping track of menstrual periods and other vaginal bleeding—a menstrual history—with the rhythm method of birth control. Indeed, that can be one of its uses. It is a mistake to think, however, that a menstrual history should be kept only by women using it for birth control. Awareness of the functioning of your body is the beginning of health maintenance. Menstruation provides many clues about the health of a woman's reproductive system. Changes or unusual irregularities in bleeding patterns require a gynecological checkup. These may be overlooked without a knowledge of your usual cycle and a record of bleeding between periods.

The method of birth control appropriate for you (see the section "Contraceptive History") may depend on your menstrual patterns: the pill is not the best method for women with highly irregular, scanty menstrual periods; the IUD may be dangerous for women with heavy, prolonged, or painful periods. Neither is to be used if you have abnormal bleeding between periods.

Some women like to know when menstruation is approaching because it helps them identify physical, psychological, and behavioral changes experienced at that time. These changes vary greatly from woman to woman, and scientific research on their prevalence, variety, and causes has only touched the surface of needed knowledge. Perhaps someday menstrual histories such as those kept in this book will be studied to help us understand these phenomena.

As you approach menopause—the end of the reproductive years—a menstrual history will help you recognize this change. Symptoms that may otherwise seem mysterious, such as hot flashes or a lack of vaginal lubrication, can be understood.

A careful menstrual history can also alert you to an unplanned pregnancy sooner than you might otherwise be aware of it, allowing you to receive early prenatal care or seek an early, safe abortion. If you want to become pregnant, a menstrual history can help you figure out the time of the cycle during which you are most likely to conceive. See the section "Natural Family Planning" (p. 147) for more details on how to determine your fertile days. A menstrual history is also a valuable diagnostic tool for women experiencing difficulty becoming pregnant.

When you are pregnant, a menstrual history is the most important factor in helping you and your practitioner anticipate your baby's expected day of arrival. A pregnancy that continues more than two weeks beyond this date can be dangerous to your unborn baby. It requires careful watching, special tests, and sometimes induction of labor. Without a record of your last normal menstrual period, it can be difficult to ascertain when this time will be reached. This is particularly true if prenatal care is sought late in pregnancy. Diagnostic tests such as a sonogram (or sound-wave picture) may become necessary. Although current medical science classifies sonograms as safe for women and fetuses, research on their long-range and possibly hidden side effects is quite incomplete. They are best avoided unless absolutely necessary.

For more detailed explanations of menstruation and female reproductive anatomy and physiology we recommend *Our Bodies, Ourselves,* by the Boston Women's Health Collective, Revised and Expanded (Simon and Schuster, New York, 1979); *A New View of a Woman's Body,* by the Federation of Feminist Women's Health Centers, (Simon and Schuster, New York, 1981); and *Womancare: A Gynecological Guide to Your Body,* by Lynda Madaras and Jane Patterson, M.D., with Peter Schick, M.D. (Avon, New York, 1981).

Your menstrual history includes a place for you to check off breast self-examination at the end of each period. This simple monthly procedure is a key factor in early detection of breast cancer, the most common type of cancer among American women. All women should practice breast self-examination, but it is particularly important for women with the following risk factors: a family history of breast cancer on your mother's side—your mother, a maternal grandmother, your sister, or mother's sister or her children (your cousins); never having had children or having had your first child after the age of thirty; early menopause or late onset of menstruation; a history of any other type of gynecologic cancer, especially cancer of the cervix, endometrium (lining of the uterus) or ovary; estrogen replacement therapy during menopause. Cystic breasts are thought to be a risk. Anyone who has had a breast biopsy (removal and examination of tissue from a breast lump) that showed cellular changes (dysplasia) is at risk for developing breast cancer. Mammograms, special X rays of the breast used to detect cancer, have been found to increase your chances of actually getting the disease, although their benefit is considered greater than this risk for women with certain other risk factors. Breast-cancer incidence increases with age; most cancers occur in women over forty. It is most common among whites, especially Europeans, and particularly Jews.

To examine your breasts, begin by looking at them in the mirror. First hold your arms at your sides, then extend them straight up, and finally place your hands on your hips and bring your elbows toward each other in front of your body. You are looking for skin changes, especially an effect where your breast skin looks like the skin of an orange. You are checking for puckering or dimpling of the skin. The breasts should look essentially the same each month; if you notice one nipple pointing in an unusual direction, this may be a danger sign.

The next step in a breast exam is to lie down with your arm over your head on the side you will examine. Use the balls of the fingers of the other hand to gently, but firmly, press all areas of the breast. One easy technique is to start at any place on the outside edge and continue around in a wide circle until you return to where you began. Then make smaller and smaller concentric circles until you come to the nipple. In this way, you won't miss any areas. Use a continuous circular motion—without removing your fingers since this might cause you to pass over some spots. When you get to the nipple, squeeze it gently; an unusual nipple discharge could signify a problem. As you bring your arm down, check underneath it, since breast tissue extends into the underarm. Repeat the procedure on the other side.

During breast exam, you may feel your ribs, especially if you are thin, breast tissue, or some cystic areas. Cysts feel lumpy and movable. Sometimes they are tender. Performing breast self-examination after your periods reduces your likelihood of feeling cysts because your hormonal levels are low at that time. During and after menopause, when your periods become irregular and finally stop entirely, you should keep this monthly record to remind yourself to do monthly breast exams. If you are confused about your findings, discuss them with your practitioner. Once you get used to what your own breasts feel like, you will be able to detect changes. You are looking for lumps, thicknesses, hardened areas.

We suggest that at your next practitioner visit you demonstrate your technique of breast self-examination so that he or she can help you learn to do it well.

MENSTRUAL HISTORY

Age at first menstrual period (menarche) _______________________________

Normal flow:

Light _______________________

Medium _______________________

Heavy _______________________

FIRST DATE OF VAGINAL BLEEDING	LAST DATE	AMOUNT OF FLOW (LIGHT, MEDIUM, HEAVY)	DESCRIBE OTHER SYMPTOMS (PAIN, CLOTS, ETC.)	BREAST SELF-EXAMINATION PERFORMED

MENSTRUAL HISTORY (continued)

FIRST DATE OF VAGINAL BLEEDING	LAST DATE	AMOUNT OF FLOW (LIGHT, MEDIUM, HEAVY)	DESCRIBE OTHER SYMPTOMS (PAIN, CLOTS, ETC.)	BREAST SELF-EXAMINATION PERFORMED
FIRST DATE OF VAGINAL BLEEDING	LAST DATE	AMOUNT OF FLOW (LIGHT, MEDIUM, HEAVY)	DESCRIBE OTHER SYMPTOMS (PAIN, CLOTS, ETC.)	BREAST SELF-EXAMINATION PERFORMED

MENSTRUAL HISTORY (continued)

FIRST DATE OF VAGINAL BLEEDING	LAST DATE	AMOUNT OF FLOW (LIGHT, MEDIUM, HEAVY)	DESCRIBE OTHER SYMPTOMS (PAIN, CLOTS, ETC.)	BREAST SELF-EXAMINATION PERFORMED

Contraceptive History

Millions of Americans use birth control. Some of these contraceptive methods are used externally and have few risks. Others—primarily for women only—work inside the body. This means that many healthy women take daily doses of medication or have foreign objects and sometimes chemicals placed inside their bodies. Many unwanted side effects of these birth-control methods are known; others may be observed as time goes on.

A birth-control method must meet personal needs. Both partners should be comfortable using it. Most important, however, it must be safe for you. When considering a method it is important to review your family and medical histories with your health practitioner to see if there are health reasons that make it a dangerous choice for you.

Whenever you see a practitioner for *any* medical problem, it is important to inform him or her of the type of birth control you use, although this information isn't always asked for. This may prevent your IUD-related infection from being misdiagnosed as appendicitis, your pill-induced headaches from being dismissed as due to tension.

It is the purpose of this section to provide you with a chart for recording the various methods of birth control that you use and any side effects that occur. Each method is briefly described and we refer you to the books listed at the end of this introduction for more detailed information. See the section "Informed Consent" (p. 116) to make sure that your rights are protected whenever you seek family-planning services.

The currently available contraceptives are the "pill" (oral contraceptives), the IUD (intrauterine device or "loop" or "coil"), and the various barrier methods: the diaphragm, the cervical cap, foam or suppositories (sometimes called by their brand names—Delfen, Emko, Encare, Semicid), and condoms ("rubbers," "prophylactics," "bags," also called by a brand name, Trojans, although there are numerous other brands). Sterilization, an operation performed on men or women, is the only *permanent* way to prevent pregnancy. It is also possible to practice birth control without the use of any artificial agents; to be effective this requires daily monitoring of your menstrual cycle and body changes that indicate fertility. See the section "Natural Family Planning" (p. 147) for more details about this method, further readings, and a sample chart to help you use it successfully.

When the pill is taken by a healthy woman for birth control, she might not consider it a medication. Yet it is a powerful drug, preventing pregnancy by its effect on the pituitary—the body's master gland. Consisting of one or two hormones—progestin and/or estrogen—the pill makes the pituitary function in some ways as if you were pregnant. Hormones that normally cause the release of the egg cell (a process called ovulation) are not secreted and pregnancy cannot occur. The lining of the uterus (the womb) continues to prepare for pregnancy each month, so you still have periods on the pill, even though no egg has been released. These periods are usually scanty and short. The pill is close to 100 percent effective if used properly, but it has many side effects. These range from the annoying, like nausea, to the life-threatening, like blood clots in the legs, heart, lungs, or brain.

Before prescribing pills, a practitioner must take a thorough family and medical history and perform a complete physical exam, including a Pap smear, a test for cervical cancer. Women who have a history of problems with blood clots (such as thrombophlebitis), strokes, coronary artery disease, liver disease, or cancer of the breast or reproductive system should never take the pill. Women with severe headaches, high blood pressure, diabetes, gallbladder disease, sickle-cell anemia, abnormal vaginal bleeding, fibrocystic breast disease or fibroadenoma, mononucleosis, leg injuries, irregular periods, heart or kidney disease should probably not use the pill. It is also a risky method for women who smoke, women over thirty-five, women suffering from depression, and breast-feeding mothers. Those with borderline high blood pressure, asthma, epilepsy, uterine fibroids, acne, varicose veins, a history of hepatitis or hair loss or facial skin discoloration (chloasma) during pregnancy should use the pill on a trial basis and discontinue it if any of these conditions worsen or occur.

All women on the pill should receive follow-up care six to eight weeks after beginning its use and at least every six months thereafter. Immediate care should be sought if any of the following danger signs are noted: swelling, tenderness, redness, warmth or pain in either leg, chest pain or difficulty breathing, headaches that won't go away, eye problems such as blurry vision, spots before your eyes or inability to see, and severe abdominal pain.

The pill affects many body functions. It may cause a reduction in certain vitamins, especially B_6 and folic acid. At the same time, it may increase the body's levels of vitamin A and a few minerals. A nutritionally sound diet is therefore important for women on the pill. We urge all women on the pill to read carefully and to use the section "Nutrition" (p. 100).

One troubling side effect of the pill is that normal periods may not return after its use is discontinued, sometimes for as long as one year. This is called post-pill amenorrhea. For a few women, periods may never return. If you stop using the pill to become pregnant, it is advisable to use a barrier method of birth control until you have a few regular periods. Use the section "Menstrual History" (p. 134) to help you keep track of these. If you should become pregnant immediately or soon after using the pill, don't forget to tell this to your practitioner on your first prenatal visit. It may affect the dating of your pregnancy, so important in assuring safe prenatal care.

The IUD is a small, plastic device inserted into the uterus after history-taking and a pelvic exam by a health practitioner. This is usually done during menstruation to avoid the risks of insertion during an early, undetected pregnancy. Scientists don't understand exactly how the IUD prevents pregnancy, although there are a number of theories. The IUD does not affect ovulation or fertilization (the meeting of the egg and sperm), but it does prevent the fertilized egg from growing into the uterus (implantation). The IUD does not prevent a pregnancy outside the uterus (an ectopic pregnancy). For this reason, women with a history of ectopic pregnancy should not use the IUD. Uterine abnormalities and abnormal vaginal bleeding also preclude its use. Because the IUD may cause an increase in menstrual bleeding and cramping, it is not the best method for women with severe menstrual cramps (dysmenorrhea), heavy periods, or anemia. Occasionally, the IUD will go through (perforate) the uterus on insertion. X rays or sonograms are then needed to locate it, and surgery is sometimes advised to remove it.

One major side effect of the IUD is an increase in your chances of developing a pelvic infection. These types of infections can be serious enough to cause permanent inability to have a child or even death. A woman with a history of such an infection should seriously consider this possibility before choosing the IUD. Women with disease involving the heart valves should not use the IUD since an infection is especially dangerous for them. Pelvic infections can be caused by gonorrhea, a type of venereal disease. All women should have a test for gonorrhea before the insertion of an IUD since it is a common disease that often shows no symptoms in women. A Pap smear for cancer should also be done. Vaginal infections and cervical inflammations should be treated before an IUD is inserted. After insertion, an IUD should be checked within three months. Subsequent visits to your practitioner should be made at least once a year.

An IUD can be spontaneously expelled by the body. This happens most often in women who have never had a child. A small IUD is better retained by them, but until recently smaller IUDs have not been as effective in preventing pregnancy. A few years ago an IUD with added copper was developed; the copper enhances its contraceptive effect so a small device can be used. Women with allergies to copper cannot use these IUDs. Copper IUDs must be changed every three years. Opinions vary as to how long other IUDs should be kept in the body, but some women use them for years without problems. This, of course, is no guarantee that a problem won't arise at any time, perhaps with little or no warning.

Danger signs in a woman using an IUD are missed periods (this could mean pregnancy; the IUD is not 100 percent effective), severe abdominal pain, fever and chills, unusual discharge from the vagina, especially with a bad odor, spotting or bleeding between periods, or extra long periods, especially if the flow is heavy with clots.

The barrier methods of birth control have fewer side effects than the pill or IUD. With proper use, they provide good protection against pregnancy. Foam and condoms, used together, approach the pill in effectiveness. These can be purchased at most drugstores without a prescription and are relatively easy to use. Instructions are provided in their packages and should be read and followed. Vaginal suppositories may be used instead of foams and are most likely similar in effectiveness, but this is still being tested. They need at least ten to fifteen minutes to dissolve in your vagina. Neither suppositories nor foam work as well alone as they do with condoms. When Encare was originally marketed in the United States in 1977, its manufacturer advertised that it was 99 percent effective; this claim has been questioned and is being investigated.

The diaphragm and cervical cap must be fitted by a family-planning practitioner. The diaphragm is a rubber cup that fits into the vagina and should not be felt when properly fitted. Used with a spermicidal jelly or cream, it must be placed inside before intercourse and removed no sooner than six hours afterwards. A diaphragm needs to be refitted after a weight loss or gain of fifteen to twenty pounds, after a pregnancy, miscarriage, or abortion. A few women cannot wear a diaphragm for anatomical reasons or because of poor muscle tone. It cannot be used by women who are allergic to rubber. Because it may press against the bladder, it should not be used by women with frequent urinary tract infections (cystitis).

The cervical cap is widely used in Europe. It is a cup, smaller than the diaphragm, which fits directly over the cervix (the neck or mouth of the womb, the entrance through which sperm must swim to meet the egg). Its advantages over a diaphragm are that it can be kept in place longer, is less messy, and can be used by women with lax muscles or urinary tract problems. It cannot be used by other women because of the size of their cervices or because of cervical infection, inflammation, or irritation, although these can be treated. Women with short fingers and long vaginas may have difficulty inserting or removing a cervical cap. The effectiveness of the cap has not been extensively tested in this country and it is not approved by the Food and Drug Administration at this time as a contraceptive method, despite its long history of successful use in Europe. Some practitioners do fit cervical caps on an experimental basis. The only way to get a cervical cap in this country is to become involved in such an experiment. If you do, you must give informed consent.

Be sure you are given the opportunity to practice insertion and removal at your first diaphragm or cervical-cap fitting. Have your practitioner check your insertion and return for a recheck one to two weeks later. If it is uncomfortable when you wear it, you can have it refitted at this visit. A yearly visit is sufficient afterwards.

Either partner can become allergic to the materials used in condoms, diaphragms, or cervical caps or to the chemicals in the various foams, suppositories, creams, or jellies. If this happens, try other brands until you find one your body tolerates.

The surest method of birth control is sterilization, although even this has its failures. It is considered a permanent method since restoring fertility after a sterilization operation is not always successful. Informed consent for sterilization must include this information. No one should ever be forced or coerced into accepting a sterilization operation. Sterilization does not interfere with sexuality. Sexual desire is not lost; men do not become impotent or stop ejaculating. Ejaculatory fluid contains everything but sperm; its amount is not decreased. Orgasm is not affected. There is no change in male or female hormones; menstruation continues normally.

The male sterilization procedure, called a vasectomy, is the cutting of the tube (vas deferens) which carries sperm to the penis in a man. The operation is done in a doctor's office although it requires a two-day rest period at home afterward. A small cut is made through the scrotum under local anesthesia, eliminating the risks involved with being put to sleep. Complications may include infection, blood clot formation, and pain or discomfort. Occasionally the procedure needs to be repeated, since the tube sometimes rejoins. It takes eight or more weeks before sterilization is actually accomplished, since sperm remain in the tube after surgery. Your practitioner must perform a sperm count before sterilization can be ascertained. Animal studies have suggested that vasectomies may result in some long-term side effects to the cardiovascular or other body systems. The evidence in humans is not conclusive to date.

Sterilization for women is done by cutting the Fallopian tubes that carry the egg to the uterus. This is called a tubal ligation. It can be done through the vagina or, more commonly, through a small incision under the navel or above the pubic bone. It may require a short hospital stay. Possible complications include damage to the bowel, bleeding, and various complications of general anesthesia. Ectopic pregnancies have occasionally followed a tubal ligation.

Many people use a variety of birth-control methods. As your life changes, so too may the method that seems most acceptable and appropriate. Use these charts to record your contraceptive use. Bring them with you, along with your family and medical histories, when you seek a new method from a practitioner. Discuss any side effects of previously used methods and benefits versus possible risks to you of the method you desire.

For more information on reproduction and birth control we recommend reading *Our Bodies, Ourselves,* Revised and Expanded, by the Boston Women's Health Collective (Simon and Schuster, New York, 1978); *Biology of Women* by Ethel Sloane (John Wiley and Sons, 1980); or *Womancare: A Gynecological Guide to Your Body* by Lynda Madaras and Jane Patterson, M.D., with Peter Schick, M.D. (Avon, New York, 1981).

Much of the information for this section is from *Contraceptive Technology 1980–1981,* 10th Revised Edition, by Robert A. Hatcher, Gary K. Stewart, Felicia Stewart, Felicia Guest, David W. Schwartz, and Stephanie A. Jones (Irvington Publishers, Inc., New York, 1980). Although this book is written primarily for health practitioners, its information is useful for anyone interested in learning more about this topic. It is not difficult to understand even without a medical background.

CONTRACEPTIVE HISTORY

Name

ORAL CONTRACEPTIVES (THE PILL)

Date began_______________ Brand________________ Dose_______________
Date discontinued_________________________ Reason_________________
Side effects or complications___________________________________

Date resumed_____________ Brand________________ Dose_______________
Date discontinued_________________________ Reason_________________
Side effects or complications___________________________________

Date resumed_____________ Brand________________ Dose_______________
Date discontinued_________________________ Reason_________________
Side effects or complications___________________________________

Date resumed_____________ Brand________________ Dose_______________
Date discontinued_________________________ Reason_________________
Side effects or complications___________________________________

INTRAUTERINE DEVICE (IUD)

Insertion date____________ Type________________ Size_______________
Date removed_____________________________ Reason_________________
Side effects____

Insertion date____________ Type________________ Size_______________
Date removed_____________________________ Reason_________________
Side effects____

DIAPHRAGM

Date fitted_______________ Type________________ Size_______________
Type of cream or jelly____
Side effects____

Date fitted_______________ Type________________ Size_______________
Type of cream or jelly____
Side effects____

Date fitted_______________ Type________________ Size_______________
Type of cream or jelly____
Side effects____

NOTES—OTHER BIRTH CONTROL METHODS AND REACTIONS

Natural Family Planning

Many women and men object to artificial methods of birth control. Some religions prohibit the use of these methods. Other objections are based on the esthetic; foam, condoms, and diaphragms may interfere with sexual pleasure for some people. Others consider them messy and annoying. Many women can't or won't risk the potential side effects of the pill or the IUD. The permanence of sterilization makes it unacceptable to most people. What choice for family planning remains when all available contraceptives are rejected?

In the past, the only natural way to practice birth control was to use the rhythm method. This involved keeping track of menstrual cycles to determine those days during each cycle when conception was possible—a woman's fertile period. Unfortunately, this method has a high failure rate. Today, thanks to increased research about the menstrual cycle, two additional ways of determining fertility are available—the cervical-mucus method and the basal-body-temperature method. The most reliable form of natural family planning involves using all of these simultaneously.

To understand how natural family planning works, you must understand fertility—the ability to become pregnant. For a woman to become pregnant, an egg cell must be released from her ovary. This process—ovulation—generally occurs once each menstrual cycle. Women ovulate twelve to sixteen days before the start of each period. But the number of days from one period until the next ovulation can vary a lot from woman to woman and from cycle to cycle. Once released, the egg cell lives for up to twenty-four hours. Sperm, however, can lie in wait for the egg for as long as three days. This means that a woman can become pregnant by having sexual intercourse on any of four or five days during each menstrual cycle. Each of the three methods of natural family planning aids in ascertaining when ovulation occurs.

Before you begin to use rhythm for birth control you must keep track of all menstrual periods for six to twelve months (see "Menstrual History" chart, p. 137). You must count the number of days in each cycle, starting with the first day of menstruation as day one. The cycle ends the day before you begin bleeding again. You use the shortest and longest cycles to figure out all of your possible fertile days. Subtracting eighteen days from your shortest cycle tells you the first possible fertile day after any period. Subtracting eleven days from your longest cycle tells you after which day you can assume you are no longer fertile in each cycle. For example, if your shortest cycle in the previous six to twelve months was twenty-five days, you must begin to abstain from sexual intercourse on the seventh day of each cycle (25 − 18 = 7). If your longest cycle was thirty-five days, you can resume intercourse after day twenty-four (35 − 11 = 24). This means you must abstain from intercourse for seventeen days. Some couples do not use rhythm to determine a period of abstinence, but to decide when to use contraceptives such as foam and condoms or a diaphragm. Of course, abstinence refers only to actual intercourse; other methods of sexual pleasure need not be avoided. Orgasm can be achieved in any way pleasurable to you as long as the penis avoids the vagina.

If your cycles are exactly the same each time, you must allow a minimum of eight possible fertile days within each cycle. This accounts for the variation in ovulation from day twelve to day sixteen. One day must then be left after day sixteen to allow for the life span of the egg. Three days must be left before day twelve to allow for the life of the sperm. Of course, the more irregular your periods, the longer your period of abstinence. Yet, even if you are faithfully abstinent, it is possible to ovulate before or after the assumed fertile period. Even women with generally regular cycles can experience unpredictable changes due to stress, fatigue, illness, or travel. This, combined with often long periods of possible fertility, account for the many rhythm-method failures.

The basal body temperature is a more accurate indicator of the occurrence of ovulation. However, it is useful only *after* you've ovulated. It can confirm the nonfertile period following ovulation but provides no indication of fertility prior to ovulation.

Basal body temperature is the body's first daily temperature before any activity is begun. This method requires careful planning. It is recommended that you use a special basal-body-temperature thermometer that clearly calibrates temperature in tenths of a degree. This can be purchased at most drugstores. The thermometer must be shaken down each night and left at your bedside, within your reach. Before getting up—even to go to the bathroom—you must take your temperature. You can record it then—or later, if you are too sleepy to read the thermometer. Ovulation is indicated by a rise of six-tenths of a degree. This can happen either sharply, in one day, or in a stepwise fashion over a few days.

The rise in basal body temperature must be sustained for three days before you can assume that the fertile period has passed. Although this may seem simple, basal-body-temperature graphs are often unclear and difficult to read. Because the increase in temperature may occur over a period of days, you do not always see a clear rise of six-tenths of a degree. You may assume that you are safe if you see three days of increased temperature of at least three-tenths of a degree higher than the preceding six days *or* four-tenths of a degree higher than the average of the preceding four days. An illness causing a fever will, of course, make your temperature charts invalid.

All this sounds terribly confusing and it can be! The basal-body-temperature method makes greater sense once you actually start to keep and interpret temperature graphs. As with the rhythm method, it is wise to keep temperature graphs for a number of months before you begin to rely on them for birth control.

The cervical-mucus method of birth control is based on the fact that normal mucus goes through characteristic changes at various times during the menstrual cycle. Right after your period, you generally have no mucus. The first mucus to appear is usually thick and sticky when tested with a finger in your vagina. This is probably not fertile mucus, but until you've become familiar with your mucus and have correlated it with your basal body temperature, it is advisable to assume that any mucus might signal fertility. Fertile mucus is wet, thin, and translucent. Just before ovulation, mucus demonstrates *Spinnbarkheit*. This means you can stretch it between your fingers into a clear, thin strand—like egg white. Remember that having sex will obscure your mucus so it is recommended that you have intercourse no more than every other night until ovulation is confirmed. (An alternative to this is to use a condom on alternate nights, if this is acceptable to you.) Vaginal infections also change your mucus. Until they are treated, you cannot use this method.

Some women experience other signs of ovulation—pain, pressure, spotting, or breast tenderness. Correlating these with cervical-mucus changes and with basal body temperature increases the accuracy of the natural method of family planning.

Some couples use the various forms of natural birth control to help with fertility. This isn't necessary when first trying to get pregnant, but it may be useful after a number of months without success. These methods are used by practitioners to help diagnose the cause of infertility.

The chart provided in this section is merely a sample of a natural-family-planning chart. Similar charts must be kept for every cycle. We do not suggest using this method without further reading and, if possible, individual counseling on its use. Many women need help interpreting their basal-body-temperature graphs before these can be effectively utilized. We recommend seeking the aid of a practitioner experienced in this method. Some Catholic hospitals offer instruction in natural family planning since it is the only method of birth control officially approved by that church. It may be referred to as the "Billings" method after Drs. John and Lyn Billings who did extensive research on cervical mucus and developed the mucus method.

As an additional resource, or if you are unable to get professional assistance, we highly recommend reading *A Cooperative Method of Natural Birth Control* by Margaret Nofziger (The Book Publishing Company, Summertown, Tenn. 1976). This simply written, beautifully designed book gives step-by-step instructions in using each of the three components of the method. It provides sample charts with interpretations of the recordings and discusses using the method during nursing, as menopause approaches, and following pill use. Unfortunately, the book may be difficult to obtain in some parts of the country. It can be ordered directly from the publisher, c/o The Farm, Summertown, Tenn. 38483. The sample chart in this section was reprinted from this book with permission of the author and The Book Publishing Company.

BASAL TEMPERATURE AND MUCUS CHART

Month_______________ thru _______________

Date																																								
Day of week M,T, W, Th, etc.																																								
Day of cycle	1	2	3	4	5	6	7	8	9	10	11	12	13	14	15	16	17	18	19	20	21	22	23	24	25	26	27	28	29	30	31	32	33	34	35	36	37	38	39	40
Temp.*																																								
.5																																								
.4																																								
.3																																								
.2																																								
.1																																								
99.0																																								
.9																																								
.8																																								
.7																																								
.6																																								
.5																																								
.4																																								
.3																																								
.2																																								
.1																																								
98.0																																								
.9																																								
.8																																								
.7																																								
.6																																								
.5																																								
.4																																								
.3																																								
.2																																								
.1																																								
97.0																																								
Mucus†																																								
Ovulation Pain Present																																								
Comment‡																																								

Number of days in this cycle: _________

*Place a dot in the center of the square under the day and across from the temperature. Connect the dots with straight lines.

†Use several descriptive words such as: creamy, wet, white, clear, sticky, slippery, spinn, milky, scant, cloudy, lots, pink, stiff, translucent.

‡Any notable circumstances: fever, illness, travel, stress, lack of sleep, emotional, etc.

Obstetrical History

An obstetrical history is a part of a woman's health history. The course of previous pregnancies, labor, and births can have significance for your current health. Most important, knowledge of past obstetrical events helps determine your chances of developing problems in subsequent pregnancies.

This section provides space for you to record the outcome of all pregnancies to date, those that ended in births as well as those that did not. Include miscarriages (spontaneous abortions), abortions, ectopic (non-uterine) pregnancies, such as tubal pregnancies, and other obstetrical complications.

We have included a place for you to record your practitioner's name and address and the hospital from which you received care during each pregnancy. You may not have known or may have forgotten details about each experience. Your present practitioner may want to get a full medical account of previous problems. Either you or your practitioner can send for your records if you know where care was given.

It may be difficult to review past disappointments and sorrows such as stillbirths. Remembrances of your original feelings may be evoked while writing this chart. We cannot reduce your pain but can only emphasize how valuable this information is to you and your practitioners. We hope you will fill out this chart completely.

BIRTHS

DATE OF BIRTH	NUMBER OF WEEKS (MONTHS)	TYPE OF DELIVERY	BABY'S INFORMATION		PROBLEMS AND TREATMENTS		PRACTITIONER & HOSPITAL NAME AND ADDRESS
			NAME & SEX	WEIGHT	MOTHER	BABY	

MISCARRIAGES (Spontaneous Abortions)

DATE	NUMBER OF WEEKS (MONTHS)	REASON (IF KNOWN)	COMPLICATIONS AND TREATMENTS	PRACTITIONER NAME AND ADDRESS	HOSPITAL

INDUCED ABORTIONS

DATE	NUMBER OF WEEKS (MONTHS)	TYPE OF ABORTION (SPECIFY— SEE LIST BELOW)	COMPLICATIONS AND TREATMENTS	PRACTITIONER NAME AND ADDRESS	HOSPITAL OR CLINIC

TYPES OF INDUCED ABORTION:

6–12 weeks (early abortion)—D & C (Dilatation and Curettage), Vacuum Aspiration (Suction)

12–18 weeks   —D & E (Dilatation and Evacuation)

16–24 weeks (late abortion)—Saline, Prostaglandins, Hysterotomy

ECTOPIC (Outside the Uterus) PREGNANCIES

Date ended		
Number of Weeks (Months)		

Location
    Tubal
    Abdominal
    Other		

Surgery Required: Removal of Pregnancy Only		
Removal of Fallopian Tube		
Removal of Tube and Ovary		
Other		
Complications		
Practitioner Name and Address		
Hospital		

MOLAR PREGNANCIES

(Hydatidiform Mole—a pregnancy in which the placenta becomes a tumor)

DATE ENDED	NUMBER OF WEEKS (MONTHS)	COMPLI-CATIONS	MEDICATIONS REQUIRED	PRACTI-TIONER NAME AND ADDRESS	HOSPITAL

4.

Childbearing

The First Experience

Reproduction is a natural part of human existence. Although we seek medical care during pregnancy, and most Americans give birth in a hospital, there is nothing abnormal about the childbearing processes. Yet, in the sections that follow, we focus somewhat on things that can go wrong—for a pregnant or postpartum woman, for a developing or newly born infant. We ask you to be aware of complications and dangers of pregnancy, labor, and delivery. We emphasize side effects of medications, environmental hazards, and illnesses of newborns. We encourage you to record your fears, frustrations, and disappointments. This is only because problems associated with reproduction experiences can importantly affect the health of mother, child, or future children. We do not intend for these pages to obscure our deeply held belief in the normalcy of childbirth and its surrounding events. As you use this section, we hope you will bear in mind that the majority of pregnancies and births occur without problems.

PREGNANCY

The relationship of a woman to her unborn child is unique within the spectrum of human relationships. When you are pregnant, anything that happens to you can potentially affect your baby—in good ways and in harmful ways. The air you breathe, the food you eat, the drugs you take, prescribed and nonprescribed, the chemicals used on your job, the pleasant and joyous moments of your life, the stresses of home, work, and perhaps even the world can all profoundly influence the growth and development of your child.

The value of keeping a pregnancy history cannot be overemphasized. We can all remember the tragic effects of the drug thalidomide on unborn children. Recently, DES (diethylstilbestrol) was found to have serious consequences for the teenaged and grown offspring of women who were given the drug to prevent miscarriage, ten, twenty, or thirty years ago. Most recently, Bendectin, a drug prescribed routinely by many practitioners for the nausea and vomiting of early pregnancy, has been called into question as a possible contributor to birth defects. The controversy looms and the investigation continues as this book goes to press.

Among the known *teratogens*—agents that cause birth defects—are viral infections such as German measles (rubella), chemicals, X rays, and many drugs, including caffeine, tobacco, and alcohol. Because our environment increasingly exposes us to such agents, we have included lists of chemical hazards and drugs commonly used in pregnancy (pp. 182 and 212). Most potential teratogens wreak the greatest havoc during the first three months or twelve weeks of pregnancy—the first trimester. This is when the baby's organ systems undergo their most intense development. For this reason, we urge women to use all drugs with caution; by the time you miss your first period, eleven to sixteen days have passed since your egg was fertilized. If you must have X rays, *always* ask for an abdominal shield. If you think you might be pregnant, postpone X rays if at all possible. Later in pregnancy, important brain development and growth occur, and preparations are made for the baby's life on the outside. He or she remains a vulnerable little creation!

One use of this section is to keep track of the many substances that may reach your baby. We have included space for you to record exposures throughout pregnancy and data about both mother and father at the time of conception. Not enough research has been done to determine how chemical exposures in a man might affect his developing child, but they are certainly worth noting. From experience we have learned the value of being diligent health historians even where the need is not immediately apparent.

Not everything a pregnant woman encounters is dangerous, of course. Fresh air, exercise, rest, and happy times may all contribute to a developing baby's well-being. Nutritious food in sufficient quantities is essential to the healthy growth of fetuses. It is recommended that an average-sized woman gain twenty-five to thirty-five pounds during pregnancy. Because we consider nutrition and exercise cornerstones of preventive health care, we have devoted separate sections to them.

Please use the sections "Nutrition" (p. 100) and "Exercise" (p. 110) along with this section for optimal health in pregnancy.

Pregnancy is certainly not a disease. Yet, to assure maternal and fetal health, care is required. We advise seeking prenatal services from an obstetrician, midwife, or family practitioner, or from a clinic specializing in these services as soon as you confirm your pregnancy. (A blood test for pregnancy can be accurate just after a menstrual period is missed; home or laboratory urine tests can usually diagnose a pregnancy two weeks after your first missed period.) Early care will help you and your practitioner anticipate problems, perform appropriate screening tests, and follow preventive measures whenever possible. In fact, it is best for a woman planning a pregnancy to have a thorough gynecological examination beforehand so that any existing problems can be treated. This exam should include blood work so that anemia can be corrected, partners can be screened if this is indicated (for example, for those with sickle-cell trait or thalessemia), genetic counseling can be initiated when necessary, and rubella vaccine can be given if you are found susceptible. In the last case, pregnancy must be postponed for three months after vaccination. A skin test for tuberculosis can be performed at this time as well so that when a chest X ray is necessary, it can be done before pregnancy.

We hope this section will serve as a guideline for evaluating the prenatal care you receive. We've indicated those tests that should be performed for all pregnant women on their first prenatal visit or soon afterward and those that should be reserved for when a problem arises. We've left space for you to keep your own record of the findings each time you see your practitioner and have provided an appropriate schedule of visits for a normally progressing pregnancy. This will let you know what each visit should consist of and will give you a continuing record of your baby's heartbeat and position, the growth of your uterus, your blood pressure, weight, the results of your urine tests, and any problems noted. We've asked you to note whether the fetal heartbeat was listened to with a special stethoscope called a fetoscope or with an instrument called a doptone which amplies the sound. This is because the doptone works on the principle of ultrasound, a type of wave whose effect on the fetus has not been thoroughly explored. Some practitioners use the doptone so that the heartbeat can be heard before the fifth month—when it can generally be picked up with a fetoscope. If the uterus is growing appropriately, however, this is not necessary. Other well-meaning practitioners use a doptone so that parents can hear the baby's heartbeat—a truly thrilling experience. With patience, however, parents can hear the heartbeat through a fetoscope. Finally, there's a place on this chart for you to list questions for your practitioner before each visit and to record danger signs that require practitioner attention. We expect this mutual communication to deepen your self-knowledge and enhance your practitioner's responsiveness to your needs.

For more information about pregnancy, we suggest the following readings:

The Pregnancy-After-30 Workbook, Gail Sforza Brewer, ed., Rodale Press, Emmaus, Pennsylvania, 1978.
Six Practical Lessons for an Easier Childbirth, Elisabeth Bing, Bantam Books, New York, 1969.
Making Love During Pregnancy, Elisabeth Bing and Libby Colman, Bantam Books, New York, 1977.
The Complete Book of Pregnancy and Childbirth, Sheila Kitzinger, Alfred A. Knopf, New York, 1980.
Right from the Start, Gail Sforza Brewer and Janice Presser Greene, Rodale Press, Emmaus Pennsylvania, 1981.

To learn more about fetal growth and development, we recommend these books:

The First Nine Months of Life, Geraldine L. Flanagan, Simon and Schuster, New York, 1962.
A Baby Is Born: The Picture Story of a Baby From Conception Through Birth, The Maternity Center Association, available from the Maternity Center Association, 48 East 92nd Street, New York, N.Y. 10028.

We also urge all pregnant women and their partners to attend childbirth-education classes. There are various methods and philosophies of childbirth education. Some classes begin early in pregnancy and prepare you for the entire experience as well as for labor and delivery. Nutrition, exercise, and relaxation are stressed. Others, starting toward the end of pregnancy, focus primarily on coping with birth itself. Breathing techniques are emphasized. Many classes incorporate postpartum care and parenting into their curriculum. For more information on classes available in your area contact the following organizations:

The American Academy of Husband-Coached Childbirth, P.O. Box 5224, Sherman Oaks, California 91413 (The "Bradley" Method of Childbirth).
American Society for Psychoprophylaxis in Obstetrics (ASPO), 1523 L Street N.W., Washington, D.C. 20005 (The "Lamaze" Method).
International Childbirth Education Association (ICEA), P.O. Box 20852, Milwaukee, Wis. 53220.
Cooperative Childbirth Network, 14 Truesdale Drive, Croton-on-Hudson, N.Y. 10520.
C/SEC, 23 Cedar St., Cambridge, Mass. 02140 (for Cesarean birth classes).

Many libraries and bookstores now have sections on health and/or pregnancy and birth. You can't possibly read too much as you attempt to develop your own philosophy and identify your personal needs.

HEALTH DATA AT TIME OF CONCEPTION

MOTHER

Age________________ Weight______________ Height______________

Occupation: Title_____________ Employer__________________ Department______________

ILLNESS(ES)

At time of conception____

Recent exposure to infection: Date__________________ Specify nature______________

MEDICATIONS TAKEN: Name__________________ Date(s)__________________
Other drug use____
Alcohol:

Type	# days per week used	# glasses per day
Beer		
Wine		
Hard Liquor		

Tobacco:	# per day
Cigarettes	
Cigars	
Pipe	

Caffeine:	# ounces or glasses per day
Colas and other sodas	
Coffee	
Tea	
Chocolate	

Pica (Unusual food cravings or ingestion of clay, dirt, ice, or laundry starch) Specify frequency and amount____
____

Date of conception, if known____

Last menstrual period: Date of first day__________________ Number of days__________________
    Amount of flow (normal/less than normal)__________________

Previous menstrual period____

Last contraceptive used: Type__________________ Date Discontinued__________________

Your calculation of your **E**stimated **D**ate of **C**onfinement (EDC) due date
    Subtract three months from the date of your last normal menstrual period and add seven days
    to the first day:____

See Medical, Obstetrical, and Family History for other relevant data.

HEALTH DATA AT TIME OF CONCEPTION

FATHER

Age_______________ Weight_____________ Height_____________

Blood type and Rh_______________________

Occupation:

Title_____________________ Employer_________________ Department_____________

ILLNESS(ES)

At time of conception____

Recent exposure to infection: Date_______________ Specify nature_____________

MEDICATIONS TAKEN:

Name_______________________________ Date(s)_______________

Other drug use_______________________

Alcohol:

Type	# days per week used	# glasses per day
Beer		
Wine		
Hard Liquor		

Tobacco:	# per day
Cigarettes	
Cigars	
Pipe	

Caffeine:	# ounces or glasses per day
Colas and other sodas	
Coffee	
Tea	
Chocolate	

Health of previous children (if any)_______________________________

See Medical, Obstetrical, and Family History for other relevant data.

RECORD OF EXPOSURES DURING PREGNANCY

List all drugs taken.
Include prescription drugs, over-the-counter drugs, legal and illegal drugs.
Include tobacco, alcohol, and caffeine.
Include even those medications that seem harmless to you, like vitamins and cold pills, aspirin, or indigestion remedies.

NAME OF DRUG	DOSAGE	REASON TAKEN	DATES TAKEN	REACTIONS

RECORD OF EXPOSURES DURING PREGNANCY

List any chemical exposures, including occupational and environmental exposures.

CHEMICAL NAME	DATE(S)	LOCATION	EXPLANATION

List all X rays, including those taken by anyone other than your prenatal practitioner or clinic. Before any X ray is taken, make sure the practitioner is informed that you are pregnant. Include dental X rays.

DATE	PART OF BODY X-RAYED	HOSPITAL OR OFFICE	PRACTITIONER	REASON

ROUTINE PRENATAL LABORATORY TESTS
(See pp. 172 to 176 for explanations.)

TEST	DATE	RESULT
Pregnancy test (urine or blood)		
Pap smear		
Gonorrhea test		
Syphilis test (VDRL, ART, or Wasserman)		
Blood type		
Rh factor		
If negative, partner's Rh factor		
Complete blood count hemoglobin		
hematocrit		
Rubella immunity screen		
Sickle screen (if appropriate: See Family History) If positive: hemoglobin electrophoresis		
Partner's sickle screen		
Partner's hemoglobin electrophoresis		
Diabetic screening test (Fasting blood sugar and/or 2-hour postprandial)		
Urinalysis		
TB Skin Test (Tine or PPD)		

SPECIAL PRENATAL LABORATORY TESTS
(See pp. 176 to 179 for explanations.)

TEST	DATES	REASON	RESULT
Chest X ray			
Sonogram (Ultrasound)			
Amniocentesis			
Glucose tolerance test (GTT)			
Rh antibody screen (If Rh negative)			
Urine Culture and Sensitivity (C & S)			
Anemia work-up			
Viral studies TORCH: *T*oxoplasmosis, *R*ubella, *C*ytomegalovirus, *H*erpes			
Nonstress test (NST) or fetal activity test (FAT)			
Oxytocin challenge test (OCT)			
Amnioscopy			
Other (specify)_____________________			

PRENATAL CARE PRACTITIONER VISITS

FIRST VISIT: Note any abnormalities on physical examination:

____

Results of clinical pelvimetry (size of pelvis):

Adequate________________   Borderline______________   Contracted____________

MONTH/WEEK (*Fill in week**)	DATE	WEIGHT	BLOOD PRESSURE	URIN-ALYSIS: GLUCOSE/ PROTEIN	SIZE/ HEIGHT OF UTERUS
2nd month ________wk					
3rd month ________wk					
4th month ________wk					
5th month ________wk					______cms
6th month ________wk					______cms
7th month ________wk					______cms
________wk					______cms
8th month ________wk					______cms
________wk					______cms
9th month ________wk					______cms
________wk					______cms
________wk					______cms
________wk					______cms
________wk					______cms
________wk					______cms
________wk					______cms

* Practitioners calculate how pregnant you are in number of weeks. Your due date is forty weeks from the first day of your last period. At each visit, ask your practitioner how many weeks you are and fill in this information.

PRENATAL CARE PRACTITIONER VISITS

DATES TO RECORD: Practitioner's Calculation of your Estimated Date of Confinement (Due Date)_______________________________________

Date of Quickening: The baby's first perceived movements. (It feels like a flutter.)_______________________________________

Suggested schedule of visits for normal pregnancy: every 4 weeks to 6 months (24 wks.); every 3 weeks to 8 months (32 wks.); every other week to nine months (36 wks.); then every week.

FETAL HEART RATE (FHR) (*Specify fetoscope or doptone*)	POSITION OF FETUS	QUESTIONS FOR PRACTITIONER PROBLEMS NOTED OR INSTRUCTIONS PROCEDURES AND TREATMENTS

COMMON COMPLAINTS OR DISCOMFORTS OF PREGNANCY

Discuss relief measures with your practitioner or childbirth educator. Many home remedies that family members or friends can recommend work quite well. However: *don't use medication without discussing it first with your practitioner and don't reduce your dietary intake of any nutrient, including salt.*

DISCOMFORT	DATE(S) NOTED
Nausea and vomiting (early in pregnancy)	
Heartburn	
Breast tenderness	
Groin ache (round ligament pain)	
Leg pains or cramps	
Feet or ankle swelling	
Vaginal discharge (note color, odor, consistency, presence or absence of itch)	
Backaches (upper, mid, lower)_______________	
Hemorrhoids	
Constipation	
Varicose veins	
Dizziness	
Nasal congestion or nosebleeds	
Painful intercourse	
Mask of pregnancy (chloasma, facial skin discoloration)	
Tingling, numbness of fingers, arms	
Shortness of breath (late in pregnancy)	

RELIEF MEASURES TAKEN

COMPLICATIONS AND POSSIBLE SIGNS OF DANGER

SYMPTOM	POSSIBLE MEANING
BLEEDING: Amount______________ Color (pink, red, brown)______________ Consistency (thick, thin, clotted, possible tissue)______________ Associated activities (sex, orgasm, activity, vaginal exam)______________	Bleeding may be caused simply by cervical irritation. In early pregnancy, it may signal a possible miscarriage. Later in pregnancy, it may be due to placental separation from the uterus (abruptio) or to a placenta that is near the cervix (previa). Both are obstetrical emergencies.
CRAMPING	In early pregnancy, may be a sign of impending miscarriage. Later it may be premature labor, practice labor, or a symptom of a urinary tract or vaginal infection.
FEVER	A sign of infection—can itself cause premature labor.
HEADACHES: severe, prolonged BLURRY VISION CHEST PAIN SWELLING: especially face and hands	All of these may be signs of toxemia, a serious disease of pregnancy which can cause convulsions if not treated.
BAG OF WATER BREAKING (leakage of fluid—indicate color: clear, yellow, or brown) ______________	May increase both mother's and baby's chance of developing an infection. Yellow or brown fluid indicates the presence of meconium, which can mean fetal distress (except in a breech).
PAIN, URGENCY, OR FREQUENCY ON URINATION	A sign of a bladder or kidney infection, which can lead to premature labor.
EXCESSIVE VOMITING	Can lead to weight loss, dehydration, and "intrauterine growth retardation" (IUGR).
LEG PAINS	Can be thrombophlebitis, a blood clot.
DECREASED FETAL MOVEMENTS FELT (Near end of pregnancy)	A clear change in baby's movement pattern—may indicate baby is having a problem or it can simply be "lightening," the baby's moving down to become "fixed" in the pelvis.

DATE(S) NOTED	DATE PRACTITIONER CONTACTED	DIAGNOSIS AND TREATMENT (IF ANY)

Routine Tests and Examinations in Pregnancy

PREGNANCY TEST

A blood or urine test can be used to confirm pregnancy. These tests look for the presence of human chorionic gonadotropin (HCG), a hormone produced only during pregnancy. A urine test is considered reliable at about six weeks after your last menstrual period. A blood test can detect HCG just after your first missed period. A urine-test kit can be purchased at many pharmacies and can be self-administered. These are generally reliable, although false positives and false negatives can occur at home or in a laboratory. An early pregnancy test can sometimes help date your pregnancy.

COMPLETE PHYSICAL EXAMINATION

Should be performed at least once in every pregnancy and should include assessment of the skin, eyes, ears, nose, throat, neck, heart, lungs, breasts, abdomen, and extremities.

PELVIC EXAMINATION

Should be performed at least once in every pregnancy, as early as possible. Should include:

Speculum Exam: a visualization of the walls of the vagina and the cervix using a metal or plastic instrument that separates the walls of the vagina. Should not be painful, although may be uncomfortable.

Bimanual Exam: an examination of the musculature of the vagina, the cervix, uterus, tubes, and ovaries with two fingers of one hand in the vagina and the other hand on the abdomen. Abnormalities, growths, pain, and tenderness should be noted. The size of the uterus should be measured.

Clinical Pelvimetry: performed during the bimanual examination, at least once in every pregnancy, this gives the examiner an estimate of the size and shape of the pelvic opening. Each of the bones of the pelvis is palpated. Results may reveal an adequate, contracted (small), or borderline pelvis. Generally, labor is permitted even if the pelvis feels small, since the size and position of the baby and the force and progress of labor are equally important in determining whether a baby can be delivered vaginally. If the pelvic cavity is small, however, labor's progress will be scrutinized more carefully. This examination is uncomfortable although not painful.

PAP SMEAR

This is a test for cancer of the cervix. A swab of cervical cells is taken during a pelvic exam and sent to a laboratory for analysis. Although a pelvic exam may be uncomfortable, the Pap smear itself is generally painless.

GONORRHEA TEST

Gonorrhea (GC) is a form of venereal or sexually transmitted disease that is quite common in this country. Untreated gonorrhea at birth can cause blindness in a baby. This painless test is done during a pelvic exam. Cells are taken from the cervix with a cotton swab and put into a special material on which the gonorrhea organisms grow. This "culture" is sent to a laboratory for a few days before growth can be evaluated.

A gonorrhea culture should be taken at least once during your pregnancy since the infection often has no symptoms in a woman. It should be repeated at any time if you believe you've been exposed to the disease (if your partner tells you that he has gonorrhea or if he has an unusual discharge from his penis). If you think you might have gonorrhea and you have had anal or oral sex, ask your practitioner to take a culture from your rectum and/or mouth.

SYPHILIS TEST (SEROLOGY)

Syphilis is another form of venereal disease. The first symptom of syphilis is a painless sore on the vagina, cervix, or penis. This sore, called a chancre, disappears without treatment. Secondary syphilis appears about six to eight weeks later. Its symptoms vary and may be as vague as a genital or body rash. These too disappear without treatment. In its long latent phase, syphilis shows no symptoms. Years later it can attack many body systems and ultimately cause death. Because a fetus can be infected with syphilis through the placenta, all pregnant women must have a blood test for the disease.

A number of laboratory methods can be used to detect syphilis in the blood, which is why the test may be called a VDRL, ART, or Wasserman. Sometimes false positives occur, so further blood studies will be performed when syphilis is suspected. Premarital blood tests are for syphilis.

BLOOD TYPE

The blood types are A, B, AB or O. This hereditary characteristic is significant if you need a blood transfusion. After you deliver, your blood type will be compared to your baby's to see if there is the possibility of any incompatibilities. These can occasionally lead to problems in newborns.

Rh FACTOR—FOR A PREGNANT WOMEN AND HER PARTNER

Rh is a blood component that is present in most people—the Rh positive—and absent in others—the Rh negative. Both are normal biologic variants. If an Rh-negative woman carries an Rh-positive child, however, serious medical problems can result. Since the Rh factor is a dominant genetic characteristic, it is possible for an Rh-negative woman's baby to be Rh positive only if her partner is Rh positive. (See the section "Family History," p. 26, for further discussion of genetics.) Your partner's blood should therefore be tested if you are Rh negative. If he too is Rh negative, you should not have problems. If he is Rh positive, your baby may be Rh positive.

Usually, mother's and baby's blood do not mix. Babies of first pregnancies are therefore usually safe from Rh disease. After birth, however, some Rh positive blood may be passed into the mother's bloodstream. She will then manufacture "antibodies" to fight the foreign Rh factor. Once manufacture begins, it can continue throughout life. In her next pregnancy, these antibodies will pass through the placenta to her baby. If that baby is Rh positive, they will attack the baby's blood. Such Rh-sensitized newborns can be quite sick.

In the past, Rh disease was not uncommon. Today, it is rare, as a result of the development of the drug RhoGAM (Rh$_o$[D]) Immune Globulin). RhoGAM is made up of antibodies against the Rh factor. If a woman receives RhoGAM after a delivery, her body will not bother to manufacture its own antibodies. The antibodies in RhoGAM are short-lived and in subsequent pregnancies the problem is avoided.

All Rh-negative women who deliver Rh-positive babies should receive an injection of RhoGAM within seventy-two hours after birth, unless they are already sensitized. It should be given after an abortion, miscarriage, amniocentesis, or an inadvertent transfusion of Rh-positive blood.

COMPLETE BLOOD COUNT (CBC)

A complete blood count (CBC) provides information about the number of red and white blood cells. Abnormalities may indicate a blood disease, anemia, or infection. Platelets, the cells necessary for blood clotting, are also measured.

Hemoglobin and hematocrit measures are part of a CBC. Hemoglobin is the oxygen-carrying chemical in the blood. Hematocrit is a measure of the percent of cells in the blood. A low hemoglobin or hematocrit signifies anemia. A CBC also gives information about the size and color of the red blood cells, useful in the evaluation of anemia.

RUBELLA IMMUNITY SCREEN

Rubella is commonly called German measles. This generally mild infection can cause serious birth defects in fetuses whose mothers are infected. Fortunately, immunity to rubella is conferred through the infection itself or the vaccine against it. This rubella test assesses immunity.

It is wise to have your immunity to rubella tested before pregnancy so that you can be vaccinated if necessary. The vaccine must be given three months before you become pregnant. If you have never had this test, pregnancy is a good time for it. It will determine your need for vaccination after pregnancy. It will also help your practitioner diagnose rubella if you are exposed to it. If you do come in contact with rubella, or develop symptoms (a rash and low-grade fever) that your practitioner suspects might be rubella, you should have a series of blood tests to see if your "titre" is rising—that is, if your body is fighting the virus by producing an increasing number of antibodies against it. If you are infected, and it is early enough in pregnancy, abortion is advised.

SICKLE-CELL SCREEN (OR SICKLE PREP)

Sickle-cell anemia is a disease of the blood's oxygen-carrying compound (hemoglobin). A sickle-cell screen is a test for sickle-cell trait or anemia. All women of African descent should be tested. If the screen is positive, a further test, called a *hemoglobin electrophoresis,* must be performed to distinguish sickle trait from sickle-cell anemia. Since this disease is inherited, if you have either the trait or the disease, your partner should be tested to determine the baby's chances of developing the disease. (See the section "Family History," p. 27.)

DIABETES SCREENING TEST: FASTING BLOOD SUGAR (FBS) AND/OR TWO-HOUR POSTPRANDIAL (2-HR. PP)

Because abnormalities in sugar metabolism—diabetes—tend to appear in pregnancy, many practitioners perform a diabetes screening test on all pregnant women. Both a fasting blood sugar (FBS) and a two-hour postprandial (2-hr. PP) assess sugar (glucose) levels in the blood. The FBS is taken after the patient has not eaten for twelve hours and the two-hour PP is taken two hours after a meal high in carbohydrates. Sometimes the patient is given a special carbohydrate mixture to drink.

Some practitioners perform one of these tests; others do both. The best time for these to be done is between twenty-eight and thirty-two weeks (the seventh month) of pregnancy. Some practitioners perform these tests only on women who are most likely to develop gestational or pregnancy diabetes. This includes women with a family history of diabetes, obese women, women who have had many pregnancies or very large babies, or who spill sugar in their urine or have persistent Monilia infections of the vagina. Excessive thirst, excessive hunger, and excessive urination are the classic symptoms of diabetes, and their presence is another indication for the test.

URINALYSIS (U/A)

Abnormalities in the urine can tell a lot about health. A urinalysis can reveal possible urinary tract infections, kidney problems, liver disorders, diabetes, dehydration (lack of sufficient fluids), starvation, or toxemia of pregnancy. A complete urinalysis should be done at least once during pregnancy. At each prenatal visit, urine should be tested for sugar (glucose) and protein (albumin). If either is present, further tests may be required to rule out diabetes or toxemia of pregnancy, respectively.

TB SKIN TEST (TINE TEST OR PPD)

TB, or tuberculosis, is a serious disease that usually attacks the lungs. Until the relatively recent development of effective treatment, TB was a major killer. The skin test consists of a shallow, pinpricklike injection into the forearm. A positive reaction, read forty-eight to seventy-two hours later, will occur if you have tuberculosis or have been exposed to it. This test should be done in pregnancy because of the seriousness of the disease to both mother and child and its contagiousness. If the skin test is positive, it must be followed by a chest X ray, although this can usually be postponed until the postpartum period. (See "Special Diagnostic Tests in Pregnancy," below.) Preventive treatment may be begun after pregnancy.

If you have ever received a tuberculosis vaccination (BCG), your skin test will show a false positive. Remember to inform your practitioner that you have been vaccinated. The vaccine has not been used in this country, but its use has been widespread in other areas such as the Caribbean.

Special Diagnostic Tests in Pregnancy

CHEST X RAY (CXR)

In the past, many practitioners ordered chest X rays routinely for all pregnant women to rule out tuberculosis. However, because of the dangers of radiation to the growing fetus, this test is now recommended only after a positive TB skin test. Even then, it is wise to wait until the postpartum period to have the X ray, unless symptoms are present or exposure is known. Never have any X rays during the first three months of pregnancy, however. If you have not had a recent TB skin test, have one before becoming pregnant. If it is positive, or if you have had a positive reaction in the past, get a chest X ray before pregnancy.

SONOGRAM (ULTRASOUND)

A sonogram is a sound-wave picture of the uterine contents. It can tell approximately how many weeks pregnant you are, how many babies are inside, how much fluid there is, where your placenta is located, and whether certain birth defects are present. In recent years, some practitioners have begun to use sonograms routinely. Research on their possible side effects to the fetus is incomplete at this time. We recommend their use only when necessary. Indications include vaginal bleeding, an excess of amniotic fluid (polyhydramnios), a uterus that is growing larger or remaining smaller than expected, or other problems in determining your due date. Women with medical or obstetrical problems may need sonograms. If your practitioner orders a sonogram for you, we suggest you discuss the reason for it.

AMNIOCENTESIS

An amniocentesis is a procedure during which a small amount of amniotic fluid is removed through a needle inserted into the abdominal wall and the uterus. It should be done with a sonogram so the placenta and baby can be located and avoided. Local anesthesia is used to minimize pain.

Examination of amniotic fluid can reveal many fetal characteristics. Certain birth defects can be detected through the fluid. If you've had a previous child with such a defect, an amniocentesis is generally advised early in pregnancy (about the fourth month). It is recommended that women over thirty-five have an early amniocentesis to rule out Down's syndrome, which becomes an increasing possibility with advanced maternal age. Amniocentesis may also be done late in pregnancy when delivery becomes necessary before term, as in cases of severe diabetes. Its purpose then is to assess the readiness of the fetus's lungs to assume their function in breathing. An amniocentesis is performed when the baby is Rh-sensitized to help determine the severity of the disease.

Amniocentesis has some risks, including fetal damage and premature labor. It should be reserved for those women who need it. Sex can be determined by an amniocentesis, but this alone is not reason enough to warrant its risks.

GLUCOSE TOLERANCE TEST (GTT)

A glucose tolerance test (GTT) is done in pregnancy when there is a strong indication of maternal diabetes or when the fasting blood sugar or two-hour postprandial is abnormal (see p. 175). A special high-carbohydrate solution is given, either by mouth or intravenously. This follows three days of a high-carbohydrate diet. Blood and urine are then tested for sugar (glucose) at intervals of one half hour, one hour, two hours, and three hours.

Rh ANTIBODY SCREEN

This blood test is for women who are Rh negative (see "Routine Tests and Examinations in Pregnancy," p. 173). It should be done periodically during pregnancy, with increased frequency as term approaches, to make sure that the mother has no Rh antibodies in her blood. If she does, an amniocentesis may be indicated to help determine the condition of the fetus.

URINE CULTURE AND SENSITIVITY (C & S)

These urine tests are done when a urinary-tract infection is suspected. A urine specimen is taken and incubated for a few days to see if bacteria grow. Heavy growth of an identifiable bacteria indicates an infection. A sensitivity test tells which antibiotics will kill the specific organism so that drugs can be prescribed appropriately.

ANEMIA WORK-UP

If you are found to be anemic and iron tablets and a diet high in iron don't help, an anemia work-up of the blood may be ordered. This consists of a group of tests to determine the type of anemia you have— pernicious anemia or B_{12} deficiency, iron deficiency or one of the anemias in which the cells destroy themselves (hemolytic anemia). Stool specimens for ova and parasites (worms) may also be ordered, especially if you have recently traveled to the tropics.

VIRAL STUDIES

Sometimes called TORCH studies for the names of the viruses *Tox*-oplasmosis, *R*ubella, *C*ytomegalovirus, and *H*erpes, these blood tests may be ordered if you have been exposed to any of these teratogenic viruses. A series of tests might be required to differentiate current from past infections. Toxoplasmosis is transmitted through cat feces and raw meat. If you have a cat, avoid contact with the feces when you change the litter. In fact, it may be wise for someone else to assume that responsibility during your pregnancy. And don't eat raw meat.

NON-STRESS TEST (NST) OR FETAL ACTIVITY TEST (FAT)

The non-stress test (NST) is used near term if fetal distress is suspected. The babies of women with medical problems such as diabetes or obstetrical problems such as toxemia should be tested. When a pregnancy goes one or two weeks beyond its due date, an NST becomes necessary. This painless test involves attaching an external electronic fetal-monitoring machine to the mother. This machine consists of two belts that go around the abdomen. One picks up uterine contractions and the other the fetal heart rate. They are attached to a recording device. A baby might be in distress if the heart rate does not speed up with fetal movement or if there are decelerations of the heart rate following any contractions that occur. (Painless contractions of the uterus do occur before labor and will be recorded by the monitor.) Further evaluation is warranted if fetal distress seems probable.

Not enough research on the effects of external fetal monitoring either before or during labor has been done to assess the potential side effects of this test.

OXYTOCIN CHALLENGE TEST (OCT)

In this test for fetal distress, uterine contractions are stimulated by the use of the chemical oxytocin. This medication is given in small amounts through an intravenous drip until contractions occur about every three minutes. If the fetal heart rate shows repeated decelerations following these contractions, fetal distress is indicated and delivery is generally called for. Possible adverse effects of this test have not been adequately studied.

RECORD OF FETAL MOVEMENT

Since decreased movements of the fetus at term may mean that he or she is in trouble, you may be asked to record the baby's movements if your pregnancy goes past your due date or if other complications arise.

AMNIOSCOPY

An amnioscopy allows your practitioner to actually see the membranes surrounding the baby. Its purpose is to assess the color of the amniotic fluid. It is done near term or when your due date has passed. If the fluid looks green or brown this indicates the presence of meconium—

the contents of the fetal bowel. It might mean the possibility of fetal distress and signals the need for further tests such as an NST or OCT. The test cannot be done if your cervix is not open (dilated) somewhat. A small cone is placed into the vagina, against the cervix, and a light is shone into it, allowing your practitioner to visualize the membranes. It is about as uncomfortable as a speculum examination.

OTHER TESTS

Diagnostic tests may be performed during pregnancy for any preexistent medical conditions, especially ones that may be aggravated by pregnancy. Examples are tests for heart function (such as EKGs) and thyroid function (T_3 and T_4, for example). Blood sugars will be carefully assessed if you have diabetes. Conditions whose symptoms are present during pregnancy may also be ruled out with various tests. A throat culture may be done, for example, if strep throat is suspected; blood tests for liver function may be ordered if you develop jaundice. Other tests may become necessary should an obstetrical complication arise. These include blood and urine chemistries for toxemia and blood-clotting studies when there is a placenta abruptio (separation of the placenta from the uterine wall), fetal death, or toxemia. New obstetrical diagnostic tests are continually being developed and perfected, such as fetoscopy, in which the fetus and bag of water are looked at through a small cut made in the abdominal wall. Whenever a test is ordered, discuss the reasons for it with your practitioner. You are entitled to informed consent (see p. 116) during pregnancy as at other times.

See "Common Diagnostic Tests" (p. 91) for more information on some of these and other tests.

The Pregnant Patient's Bill of Rights

The Pregnant Patient has the right to participate in decisions involving her well-being and that of her unborn child, unless there is a clearcut medical emergency that prevents her participation. In addition to the rights set forth in the American Hospital Association's "Patient's Bill of Rights" (which has also been adopted by the New York City Department of Health), the Pregnant Patient, because she represents TWO patients rather than one, should be recognized as having the additional rights listed below.

1. *The Pregnant Patient has the right,* prior to the administration of any drug or procedure, to be informed by the health professional caring for her of any potential direct or indirect effects, risks or hazards to herself or her unborn or newborn infant which may result from the use of a drug or procedure prescribed for or administered to her during pregnancy, labor, birth or lactation.
2. *The Pregnant Patient has the right,* prior to the proposed therapy, to be informed, not only of the benefits, risks and hazards of the proposed therapy but also of known alternative therapy, such as available childbirth education classes which could help to prepare the Pregnant Patient physically and mentally to cope with the discomfort or stress of pregnancy and the experience of childbirth, thereby reducing or eliminating her need for drugs and obstetric intervention. She should be offered such information early in her pregnancy in order that she may make a reasoned decision.
3. *The Pregnant Patient has the right,* prior to the administration of any drug, to be informed by the health professional who is prescribing or administering the drug to her that any drug which she receives during pregnancy, labor and birth, no matter how or when the drug is taken or administered, may adversely affect her unborn baby, directly or indirectly, and that there is no drug or chemical which has been proven safe for the unborn child.
4. *The Pregnant Patient has the right,* if Cesarean birth is anticipated, to be informed prior to the administration of any drug, and preferably prior to her hospitalization, that minimizing her and, in turn, her baby's intake of nonessential preoperative medicine will benefit her baby.
5. *The Pregnant Patient has the right,* prior to the administration of a drug or procedure, to be informed of the areas of uncertainty if there is NO properly controlled follow-up research which has established the safety of the drug or procedure with regard to its direct and/or indirect effects on the physiological, mental and neurological development of the child exposed, via the mother, to the drug or procedure during pregnancy, labor, birth or lactation—(this would apply to virtually all drugs and the vast majority of obstetric procedures).
6. *The Pregnant Patient has the right,* prior to the administration of any drug, to be informed of the brand name and generic name of the drug in order that she may advise the health professional of any past adverse reaction to the drug.
7. *The Pregnant Patient has the right* to determine for herself, without pressure from her attendant, whether she will accept the risks inherent in the proposed therapy or refuse a drug or procedure.
8. *The Pregnant Patient has the right* to know the name and qualifications of the individual administering a medication or procedure to her during labor or birth.

9. *The Pregnant Patient has the right* to be informed, prior to the administration of any procedure, whether that procedure is being administered to her for her or her baby's benefit (medically indicated) or as an elective procedure (for convenience, teaching purposes or research).

10. *The Pregnant Patient has the right* to be accompanied during the stress of labor and birth by someone she cares for, and to whom she looks for emotional comfort and encouragement.

11. *The Pregnant Patient has the right* after appropriate medical consultation to choose a position for labor and for birth which is least stressful to her baby and to herself.

12. *The Obstetric Patient has the right* to have her baby cared for at her bedside if her baby is normal, and to feed her baby according to her baby's needs rather than according to the hospital regimen.

13. *The Obstetric Patient has the right* to be informed in writing of the name of the person who actually delivered her baby and the professional qualifications of that person. This information should also be on the birth certificate.

14. *The Obstetric Patient has the right* to be informed if there is any known or indicated aspect of her or her baby's care or condition which may cause her or her baby later difficulty or problems.

15. *The Obstetric Patient has the right* to have her and her baby's hospital medical records complete, accurate and legible and to have their records, including Nurses' Notes, retained by the hospital until the child reaches at least the age of majority, or, alternatively, to have the records offered to her before they are destroyed.

16. *The Obstetric Patient,* both during and after her hospital stay, has the right to have access to her complete hospital medical records, including Nurses' Notes, and to receive a copy upon payment of a reasonable fee and without incurring the expense of retaining an attorney.

It is the obstetric patient and her baby, not the health professional, who might sustain any trauma or injury resulting from the use of a drug or obstetric procedure. The observation of the rights listed above will not only permit the obstetric patient to participate in the decisions involving her and her baby's health care, but will help to protect the health professional and the hospital against litigation arising from resentment or misunderstanding on the part of the mother.

Prepared by Doris Haire, Chair., Committee on Health Law and Regulation, National Women's Health Network. Reprinted with Permission.

ENVIRONMENTAL EXPOSURES AFFECTING REPRODUCTION
By Judith Greenberg

OCCUPATIONAL HAZARDS WITH KNOWN OR SUSPECTED EFFECTS ON REPRODUCTION	
VINYL CHLORIDE (VC)	Documented carcinogen, linked to angiosarcoma of the liver; implicated in chromosomal aberrations of male germ cells; with increased miscarriage rate and birth defects in humans.
CHLOROPRENE	Chemically related to vinyl chloride; functional disruption of spermatogenesis found in exposed males; studies show threefold increase in miscarriage rate among their wives.
BENZENE	Prolonged menstrual periods, associated with aplastic anemia and leukemia; associated with chromosomal aberrations.
TOLUENE	Derivative of benzene, less toxic; associated with chromosomal aberrations.
XYLENE	Derivative of benzene; causes birth defects in chicks.
CADMIUM	Implicated in bronchogenic and prostatic cancer; in animal tests caused damage to testicular tissue; sterility in test animals, teratogenic effects, low birth weights; heavy smoking increases the risk—cigarette smoke high in cadmium.
LEAD	Studies on human populations, associated with sterility, menstrual disorders, birth defects, prematurity, mental retardation and chromosomal aberrations.
MERCURY	CNS damage in humans, cerebral palsy type symptoms in exposed infants from studies in Minnimata, Japan; behavioral alterations in animal offspring.
CARBON TETRACHLORIDE	Suspected carcinogen, passes through placenta and causes fetal liver damage in animals; specific toxicity to liver and kidneys.
TRICHLORETHYLENE (TCE)	Can damage liver and kidneys, suspected carcinogen; no studies of genetic risks done.
PERCHLORETHYLENE	Acts similarly to TCE; carcinogenic studies not completed.
POLYCHLORINATED BIPHENYLS (PCBs) (CHLORINATED DIPHENYLS)	Liver cancer and reduced fertility in animals; "cola colored babies" in Japan with high frequency of growth retardation, gingival hyperplasia, spotted skull calcification; studies show accidental oral intake can be embryotoxic, causing stillbirths.

NITROSAMIDES	These compounds can induce nervous system tumors in up to 100 percent of the offspring when mother animals are injected on the fifteenth day of pregnancy.
CARBON DISULFIDE	Menstrual irregularities, decreased fertility and frequent miscarriages in women; decreased libido and sperm abnormalities reported in men.
BIS (CHLOROMETHYL) ETHER	Known human carcinogen; combination of formaldehyde and HCL in warm, moist air can form BIS ether; possible effects on the fetus should be considered.
RADIATION	Ionizing radiation associated with chromosomal aberrations, increased sterility, and birth defects; children prenatally exposed have two times the rate of leukemia; Czech study implicates microwave/RF (radio frequency) radiation with retarded fetal development, congenital defects, increased miscarriage rate; animal studies show teratogenic effects.
MANGANESE	Impotence and decreased libido in exposed males.
ESTROGENS	Heavier and more frequent menses, increased incidence of birth defects (teratogenic), and carcinogenic (DES) in offspring; male workers—enlarged breasts and increased impotency.
PESTICIDES CHLORINATED HYDROCARBONS	All have been implicated in causing cancer; kepone can cause sterility in males and decreased libido; animal studies show increased abnormalities in offspring and increased infertility in female animals.
CARBON MONOXIDE	Chronic exposure caused decreased birth weight and increased neonatal mortality in rats; acute exposure has caused fetal and combined fetal-maternal deaths.

JOBS COMMONLY HELD BY WOMEN AND THE POTENTIAL HAZARDS

OCCUPATION	POTENTIAL HAZARD

HOSPITAL WORKERS
  RNs
  NURSES' AIDES
  ANESTHETISTS
  LAB WORKERS
  DENTAL ASSISTANTS
  MDs
  DENTISTS, ETC.
	*X rays
	*radioisotopes
	infectious diseases
	anesthetic gases
	ozone
	formaldehyde
	*benzene
	toluene
	ethylene oxide
	mercury
	volatile organic compounds
	hexachloroprene
	*BIS (chloromethyl ether)

CLERICAL WORKERS	ozone (copying machines) spores, dust *asbestos *benzene toluene *trichlorethylene ("white out" and "cleaners")
LAUNDERING AND DRY CLEANING	infectious and chemical contamination from clothing *trichlorethylene perchlorethylene petroleum solvents (naphtha) *benzene soaps, detergents, bleaches *carbon tetrachloride
TEXTILE AND APPAREL	*benzene toluene *dyes, aniline cotton dust *asbestos formaldehyde *trichlorethylene perchlorethylene *chloroprene styrene carbon disulfide
ELECTRONIC WORKERS RUBBER WORKERS	terrulium *nitrosamides *trichlorethylene chloroform acetone sulfuric acid *arsenic *lead microwave radiation zinc

ELECTRONIC WORKERS RUBBER WORKERS (*cont.*)	*polychlorinated biphenyls (PCBs) mercury
AGRICULTURAL WORK MEAT HANDLERS	*pesticides, all types *chloroprene anthrax brucellosis

OUTDOOR WORK
  TOLL BOOTH OPERATORS
  TRAFFIC CONTROL
  AIRLINE STEWARDESSES
	carbon monoxide

HAIRDRESSERS AND COSMETOLOGISTS	*hair dyes nail sprays—monothanolamine nail varnishes plasticizers benzyl alcohol ethyl alcohol acetone xylene toluene *benzene depilatories—sodium thioglycolate permanent wave solutions ammonium thioglycolate *asbestos in hair dryers *vinyl chloride hair spray propellant

ARTS AND CRAFTS
  PAINTERS
  PRINTERS
  STAINED-GLASS WORKERS
  POTTERS
  SILK-SCREEN MAKERS
  WOODWORKERS, ETC.
	*benzene
	toluene
	*lead
	silica
	mineral spirits
	turpentine
	mercury
	lithium and barium
	epoxy resins
	methylene chloride
	*benzidine derivative dyes
	spray polyurethane foams
	*chromium

* Confirmed or suspected occupational carcinogens.
From the *Journal of Nurse-Midwifery*, Vol. 25, No. 4, July/August 1980. Reprinted with Permission.

PREGNANCY DIARY

Pregnancy is a time of awesome biologic events, many incompletely understood. The incredible physical changes that create a new life and an environment specialized to ensure its survival are perhaps matched only by the psychological and emotional impact of the experience.

Nature seems to have provided a useful psychological mechanism to enable women to appreciate this part of their lives—the increasing self-involvement and introspection that so many women feel as pregnancy advances. Yet, in our busy, business- and production-oriented society, the time just to sit and think has become a rare privilege for most of us. Other children call us with their never-ending needs. The daily work of earning a living, coupled with household tasks, leave most of us with all too few leisure hours to be alone or to share special moments with loved ones.

With pregnancy comes also a sense of responsibility to the unborn. We sense that this new life should be protected—from environmental hazards and pollutants, from tension, from whatever hardships we adults face. This is not merely a romantic notion indulged in by a pregnant woman—it is a genuine need of the fetus. Medical science has discovered that the placenta, the source of the baby's nourishment and oxygen and his or her link with mother-to-be, is not the barrier it was previously considered. Almost everything a pregnant woman eats, smokes, inhales, absorbs, and secretes within her own body affects her baby.

The practical, the economic, the personal upheavals of our lives, the unavoidable problems we face at home and at work all create emotional stress to which the body responds. During this "fight or flight" response, there is an increase in the body of a group of chemicals called catecholamines. It is known that these chemicals can alter the blood supply to the fetus, but how this might affect a growing baby is not exactly known. Yet few, if any, women experience pregnancy without emotional upsets, even conflicting feelings about the pregnancy itself.

We suggest that you use these pages to record the emotional experiences of pregnancy. Keep track of the stressful as well as the positive feelings—perhaps this may even help work them out. You can't always change the conditions of your life, but you can express your feelings and use this expression to ease some of the tension. Vivid dreams are common in pregnancy. Record them here—the fearful and the happy—with your fantasies and your realities. The literature of pregnancy remains to be written; perhaps it will evolve from pages such as these. We also encourage sharing these feelings with others—your partner, your mother, sisters, friends who have themselves experienced pregnancy, coworkers who share job frustrations.

For helpful reading on the emotional aspects of pregnancy for parents-to-be, see *Pregnancy: The Psychological Experience* by Arthur and Libby Colman (Bantam Books, New York, 1971) and *The Experience of Childbirth* by Sheila Kitzinger (Pelican Books, Gretna, Louisiana, 1967).

PREGNANCY DIARY

Second Month

Third Month

Fourth Month

Fifth Month

PREGNANCY DIARY *(continued)*

Sixth Month

Seventh Month

Eighth Month

Ninth Month

LABOR AND DELIVERY

Whoever gave labor its name was a wise person indeed. Giving birth is very likely the most difficult work a human being can do. The process can be slow, painful, exhausting, at times frustrating and frightening. It is truly an altered state of consciousness, one that drastically changes a woman's relationship to her body. With thoughtful preparation and loving support, however, the accomplishment of labor can be a source of great personal satisfaction. It can inspire fascination with nature's workings and respect for the body's ability to reproduce itself in minute detail. The mystery of labor does not create this wonder; rather, an understanding of the process makes us appreciate it.

A number of events must occur in labor. The cervix or mouth of the womb (uterus) must thin (efface) and open (dilate) to permit the baby to enter the world. The baby must leave the uterus and descend into the birth canal—the vagina. These three tasks—effacement, dilatation, and descent—are accomplished by the force of intermittent contractions of the muscles of the uterus. These contractions cause the pain of labor.

Labor has been divided into three stages. The first or dilation stage begins with the beginning of contractions and ends in complete opening of the cervix; the second or pushing stage ends with the birth of the baby, and the third or placental stage ends with the birth of the placenta (afterbirth). Exactly why and how labor begins remains a question for scientific research.

How well labor proceeds depends upon the strength and pattern of the contractions, your general health, prior to and during labor, the size and position of your baby, the size and shape of your pelvis, and the environment in which you labor. Your emotional well-being plays a significant part in the progress of labor. Relaxation can facilitate labor, tension impede it. Medications can foster relaxation but can also prolong labor. The presence of a familiar person can not only make labor easier to tolerate but can actually shorten it. We firmly believe that no one should *ever* be without support in labor. Even the most compassionate medical and hospital personnel cannot replace friends, lovers, family members. Besides these identifiable factors, labor is undoubtedly influenced by many as yet unknown.

Labor is a time of uncertainties. How long it will take, how much endurance it will require, and how normally it will proceed are never entirely predictable. The vast majority of labors, of course, are normal and produce healthy infants. Careful prenatal screening can determine the likelihood of serious complications arising during any labor. The criteria used are based on your medical and family histories, history of the pregnancy and of previous pregnancies, labors, and births, and health of other children.

Problems during labor can affect you or your baby or both. Labor itself can fail to progress; the baby may be too large to pass through the pelvis; mothers may develop fatigue, dehydration, infection, or toxemia (a serious disease of pregnancy that can lead to seizures if untreated). Hemorrhaging, during or after labor, is possible. For full-term babies, normal labor and birth pose no problems. In fact, it is thought that they provide valuable stimulation to help in the baby's immediate adjustment to life outside the womb. Babies whose mothers have medical problems such as diabetes or obstetrical problems such as toxemia may have a difficult time enduring birth's hardships, however. Premature babies, babies in unusual positions, such as feet or buttocks first (breech), babies already sick, such as those with the now-rare Rh disease, are also at risk.

To protect your health and that of your baby, the labor experience must be a closely monitored one. Choice of the birthplace should be based on personal preference and identified maternal and fetal risk factors. A large medical complex is generally best if you have any problems or if any are anticipated. A birth in a birthing center or at home may be chosen by families without risk factors. A community hospital may be the place of choice for women with no or few risks who prefer a hospital, or for women with problems if a large medical complex is inaccessible. Careful observations must be made wherever you labor by practitioners experienced in caring for laboring women.

During labor, your temperature, pulse, respiratory rate, and blood pressure should be followed; you should be given lots of fluids—to drink if possible; if you cannot drink, you may need an intravenous drip. You should be assisted to walk unless there are risk factors, such as increased blood pressure, that require rest, medication, or special equipment for monitoring you or your baby. Babies who are experiencing difficulty sometimes pass meconium—the greenish-brown contents of the fetal bowel. Therefore, when the bag of waters breaks (called "rupture of the membranes"), evaluating the color of the fluid is important. The baby's heart must be listened to quite often with a special stethoscope called a fetoscope or it must be continuously picked up with an electronic fetal-monitoring machine. The monitor is a helpful tool for babies at risk but should never replace one-to-one contact with nursing and medical staff. When an abnormal heart-rate pattern is perceived, a sample of the baby's blood, taken directly from his or her scalp, can indicate whether the baby is in trouble. Serious fetal distress signals the need for rapid delivery of the baby since it can result in breathing difficulties at birth and possibly lead to permanent damage of the central nervous system. There is evidence that events in labor may contribute to such problems as learning difficulties caused by minimal brain damage. If a distressed baby is not ready to be born spontaneously, a forceps or vacuum delivery may be advised if you are fully dilated and the baby has descended enough; otherwise a Cesarean birth may be necessary.

During labor a fetus is quite susceptible to the effects of substances given to you. These can depress the baby directly or affect your circulatory system in such a way that the baby's oxygen supply is reduced. Generally, medications given to women in small doses at the appropriate time before birth don't produce serious effects on the baby, but subtle effects on development are suspected by some experts.

Narcotics and tranquilizers such as Demerol and Phenergan are often used to treat the pain and anxiety of labor. Anesthesia to numb the lower part of the body (epidural, caudal, spinal) is another common method of pain relief. This involves injecting medication through a small tube placed into or below the spinal canal. Other medications may be given in labor when a mother is ill. An example of this is magnesium sulfate for toxemia. Medications may also be given to stop premature labor or to help mature a premature baby's lungs to prevent "respiratory distress syndrome" after birth. Labor can be started (induced) or aided (stimulated) with a medication called Pitocin. Pitocin is the brand name of a manufactured form of oxytocin; oxytocin is the same hormone that the body produces in labor. The Food and Drug Administration has forbidden the use of Pitocin for induction of labor for convenience; it can only be used when there is a problem necessitating delivery. Any time a medication is given, you and your baby require constant supervision.

Some medications are given only in the second stage of labor, just for birth. Sometimes a forceps delivery requires that you be put to sleep with general anesthesia. This is occasionally also necessary for other complications such as a retained placenta. Other birth medications are given to numb the perineum—the area between the vagina and anus. This is the part of the body that must stretch to allow the vagina to open enough to permit passage of the baby. Numbing is sometimes needed to cut and always to repair an episiotomy, when one is called for. An episiotomy is the small incision made into the perineum when it won't stretch enough on its own. This cut may be made in the middle, extending from the vagina to above the anus (a median episiotomy) or it may be off to one side (mediolateral episiotomy). At times, the vagina or perineum will tear on its own. These lacerations can be superficial or deep (first or second degree) or even include the anus and possibly rectum (third or fourth degree). The numbing medication—lidocaine—is similar to that used by a dentist. It can be injected directly into the skin and underlying tissue (local anesthesia) or into a nerve that passes through the vagina and controls sensation in the area (pudendal block anesthesia). Generally, these are considered safe unless you have an allergy to the medication or unless it is used in too great a quantity or accidentally injected into a blood vessel.

Beyond the basic safety factors outlined in this section, the way labor and delivery is viewed and treated has become the source of impassioned debate and disagreement. The issues focus on the questions of intervention in nature's processes and control of the experience. On one side of the intervention question are those who advocate aggressive use of medical procedures and technology. They believe all fetuses should be monitored with electronic fetal monitors. Such practitioners keep mothers in bed to facilitate monitoring; they use intravenous rather than oral feedings just in case a Cesarean section should become necessary. Interventionists tend to break the bag of waters artificially if it doesn't break on its own. The rationale for this action varies, but includes the need to monitor the baby's heartbeat through an electrode placed directly on its scalp, the possibility of speeding up labor, and the value of seeing if meconium is present.

The opponents of such interventions point out that they are unnecessary for most mothers and babies and that the use of technology increases depersonalization of care. More important, they argue that intervention creates its own problems. Scalp electrodes can cause abscess formation; rupturing the bag of waters can cause labor to be more traumatic for the baby and possibly increase chances of infection; injudicious use of fetal monitors can contribute to an increase in the number of Cesarean sections performed, with their attendant risks for women. Supporters of the less-interventionist philosophy believe that the family has the right to decide, on the basis of informed consent, what procedures they want in childbirth, barring an emergency situation. Besides those mentioned, such procedures include routine repeat Cesarean sections, without providing a chance for labor, routine use of enemas, shaves, intravenous drips, episiotomies, delivery-room tables with stirrups for birth, and separation from the newborn. One result of this conflict has been the development of a national network of out-of-hospital birthing centers and a strong movement for home birth.

We believe in individualized care for all families, based on standards of safety and personal decision-making. We have included with these charts a checkoff list of those practices you may or may not want for your birth experience. We thank Suzanne Arms and Don Creevy, who prepared this Birth Plan, for allowing us to reprint it. We suggest reading more about the processes of labor and birth to help decide what your own values and beliefs are. Discuss your feelings with your practitioner or the practitioners in your clinic. Assess your potential risk factors together. If you feel you have important disagreements that cannot be resolved by discussion, we suggest changing practitioners or clinics.

Most of the books listed in the section "Pregnancy" discuss labor and delivery as well. In addition, we suggest the following:

> *Spiritual Midwifery,* Ina May Gaskin, The Book Publishing Company, The Farm, Summertown, Tenn., 1978 (available from the publisher).
>
> *The Cesarean Birth Experience,* Bonnie Donovan, Beacon Press, Boston, 1978.
>
> *Birth in Four Cultures: A Cross-Cultural Investigation of Childbirth in Yucatan, Holland, Sweden and the U.S.,* Bridgitte Jordan, Eden Press Women's Publications, Inc., Montreal, 1978.
>
> *Immaculate Deception: A New Look at Childbirth in America,* Suzanne Arms, Houghton Mifflin Company, Boston, 1975; Bantam Books, New York, 1977.
>
> The following four books are published by the National Association of Parents and Professionals for Safe Alternatives in Childbirth and are available from NAPSAC Publications, P.O. Box 267, Marble Hill, Mo. 63764.
>
> *Safe Alternatives in Childbirth,* David Stewart and Lee Stewart, eds., 1976.
>
> *21st Century Obstetrics Now!* Volumes 1 & 2, David Stewart and Lee Stewart, eds., 1977.
>
> *Compulsory Hospitalization or Freedom of Choice in Childbirth?* Volumes 1, 2 & 3, David Stewart and Lee Stewart, eds., 1979.
>
> *The Directory of Alternative Birth Services and Consumer Guide,* Braun, Buttons, Simkin and Stewart, eds., 1980.

BIRTH PLAN

Name____

Due Date (if applicable)________________________________

BEGIN TO DESIGN YOUR BIRTH by choosing which of the following possible practices and procedures you would like to include in the experience. Assume that there will be no overriding medical or legal necessity for or against any of them in your individual case. Answer YES or NO or leave BLANK if you have no preference one way or the other.

PREPARATION

__________ enema __________shave/prep

__________ mini-prep

__________ hospital gown (instead of own clothing)

__________ intravenous drip in labor

__________ consent to be a teaching patient (Students and staff may be present at any time.)

Other____

LABOR

__________ food/fluids on request throughout labor

__________ external electronic fetal monitoring *throughout* labor

__________ external electronic fetal monitoring *for test strip only*

__________ internal electronic monitoring (This requires rupture of membranes and attachment of electrode to baby's scalp *in utero.)*

__________ monitoring baby's heart by hand fetoscope

__________ one-to-one nursing support and care during labor

__________ freedom to choose positions and activity in labor (walking, sitting, squatting, lying on side, etc.)

__________ vaginal examination for specific medical indication only

__________ lying in bed during labor

__________ full information on risks and benefits of each suggested medical procedure

__________ artificial rupture of membranes

__________ artificial hormone (Pitocin typically) to boost contractions or induce labor

__________ analgesia or anesthesia for pain in labor

kind preferred__________________________

__________ mate/chosen person present from entry to hospital through labor

__________ mate/chosen person present during any medical procedure

__________ admission papers completed in mother's room

__________ continuous labor support by person(s) in addition to mate

__________ siblings present for labor

__________ presence of translator

language_______________________________

Other____

BIRTH

__________ presence of mate/chosen person during actual birth

__________ presence of other chosen person(s) during actual birth (in addition to hospital team)

Who_______________________________________

__________ siblings present for birth

__________ mate/chosen person present for any Cesarean

__________ birth and recovery in same room as labor

__________ position in pushing phase and at delivery chosen by mother (sitting, hands and knees, side, etc.)

__________ pushing begun upon mother's urge, after dilatation complete

__________ episiotomy

__________ freedom to touch baby during delivery

__________ father/mother assisting with actual delivery by hand

__________ midwife attending

__________ physician attending

__________ female rather than male physician

__________ delivery room warmed for birth above 70°

BIRTH PLAN (continued)

___________ dimmed lights for actual birth

___________ no mask worn by father during birth (to enhance contact with baby)

___________ baby allowed to take first breaths unassisted (no immediate suctioning, etc.)

___________ late cord clamping (after pulsating stops)

___________ skin-to-skin contact with baby immediately after birth for mother and father

___________ baby cleaned before presenting to mother

___________ artificial hormone injection after delivery to contract uterus and expel placenta

___________ baby on breast (nipple stimulation) to contract uterus and expel placenta

___________ electronic warmer for baby

___________ Leboyer bath

___________ silver nitrate delayed at least one hour (for eye contact)

___________ vernix (creamy secretion on skin at birth) left on

___________ baby weighed, measured, footprinted in parents' presence after initial bonding time between parents and baby

Other___________________________

RECOVERY

___________ separate recovery area for mother while baby goes to nursery

___________ recovery with baby in privacy

___________ presence of mate/person(s) of choice with mother in recovery

Other___________________________

POST-RECOVERY

___________ baby remains in nursery except for feedings

___________ modified rooming-in

___________ baby remains with mother at all times (nights included)

___________ nurse available on request during postbirth stay

___________ person of choice in mother's room at any time of day

___________ sibling(s) visitation with mother in maternity

___________ sibling(s) visitation in mother's room with baby

___________ breast-feeding on demand from birth

___________ help with breast-feeding on request (from skilled person)

The Birth Plan is reprinted with permission from its coauthors, Suzanne Arms and Don Creevy, M.D. The original is part of the handbook from the film *Five Women, Five Births: A Film About Choices and Decisions* by Suzanne Arms. For more information write Suzanne Arms Productions, 151 Lytton Avenue, Palo Alto, California 04301.

BIRTH PLAN FOR UNEXPECTED SITUATIONS

This plan outlines some situations that you may unexpectedly encounter during your birth experience. Even when complications do arise, you can choose practices and procedures that you would like, barring further complications and problems. For some of these situations, you may not, of course, be able to predict how you will feel and you may choose to postpone your decision until the time comes, or you may find yourself changing your decision based on immediate feelings. We want you to be aware, however, of the variety of circumstances about which you can and should have input in decision-making. We thank Suzanne Arms for suggesting that readers think about decisions beyond those suggested in her original Birth Plan.

CESAREAN BIRTH
__________ epidural or spinal anesthesia (to be awake)
__________ general anesthesia (to be asleep)
__________ mate/chosen person to wait outside delivery room
__________ mate/chosen person present for Cesarean
__________ only if mother awake
__________ if mother awake or asleep
__________ to see baby in delivery room
__________ to hold baby in delivery room
__________ to breast-feed baby in delivery room
__________ father or chosen person to see and hold baby in delivery room or outside delivery room

__________ trial of labor for breech
__________ bikini incision (if possible)
__________ trial of labor for next birth (requires "transverse" or "low-flap" incision into uterus—usually possible)

CESAREAN BIRTH—POSTPARTUM
__________ rooming with another Cesarean-birth mother
__________ baby remains in nursery except for feedings
__________ rooming-in with baby
__________ modified, daytime only
__________ with IV
__________ only after IV removed
__________ complete, 24-hour
__________ with IV
__________ only after IV removed

NEWBORN WITH PROBLEMS
__________ to be taken to newborn nursery to see baby immediately
__________ with IV and Foley catheter (urinary collecting tube)
__________ only after IV and/or Foley removed
__________ to breast-feed, even if need to pump breasts while baby can't take breast
__________ to breast-feed only if baby can take breast from birth
__________ to touch baby, even if in isolette (incubator)
__________ to participate in baby's care
__________ only holding and feeding
__________ to be taught some nursing-care procedures

NEWBORN WITH PROBLEMS WHO REMAINS IN HOSPITAL AFTER MOTHER IS HOME
__________ to have access to baby at all times, for mother and father
__________ to continue to pump breasts
__________ to bring breast milk to baby to feed
__________ to participate in care

RECORD OF LABOR

Due Date _______________________   Support Person(s) _______________________

Date of Labor _______________________   Number of weeks pregnant _______________________

LENGTH OF LABOR

First stage (dilatation)   _______________

Second stage (pushing)   _______________

Third stage (placental)   _______________

MEDICATIONS USED (See chart of Commonly Used Medications in Labor, pp. 214–216)

REASON	MEDICATION	DOSAGE/ NO. TIMES GIVEN	HOW GIVEN (BY MOUTH, INTRAVENOUSLY, BY INJECTION)
For induction of labor			
For stimulation of labor			
For sleep in early labor			
For pain relief (analgesia)			
For relaxation			
For episiotomy repair			
For medical or obstetrical problem(s) (Specify problem[s]) _______			
For anesthesia			
If premature, medications used to stop labor			
If premature, medications given to mature baby's lungs			
Other (Specify)			

If labor was induced or stimulated, give reason_______________________________

If other medications were given, give reason_________________________________

Was electronic fetal monitor used? (Specify brand name of machine used.)__________
  Reason____
    Internal: For fetal heart rate   _______________________
               For uterine contractions   _______________________
    External: For fetal heart rate   _______________________
               For uterine contractions   _______________________
Was blood sample taken from baby?__________
Was scalp pH done?__________________   Number of times______________
Reasons_____________________________   Results______________________

X RAYS

How many were taken?____
Reasons: 1. to assess size of pelvis (pelvimetry)______________________
          2. to assess position of baby____________________________
          3. other (specify)_____________________________________

BAG OF WATERS

  Did bag of waters break spontaneously, or was it broken by obstetrician or
midwife?____
  Before labor?____________________   During labor?_______________
  Color of fluid?____________________   Specify number of cms:_________
  Meconium?______________________

COMPLICATIONS OF LABOR—SPECIFY AND DESCRIBE

RECORD OF DELIVERY

TYPE OF DELIVERY
Normal spontaneous vaginal (NSVD) ___________________________

Forceps (specify low or mid) ___________________________

Vacuum ___________________________

Cesarean section (specify classical or transverse) ___________________________

Breech (specify spontaneous, assisted, breech
extraction) ___________________________

ANESTHESIA USED
Specify type (see chart, p. 216) ___________________________

PERINEUM
Was episiotomy done? ___________________________

Type: Median ___________________________

Mediolateral (left or right) ___________________________

Laceration:
1st degree (involving skin only or vaginal tissue) ___________________________

2nd degree (involving muscle) ___________________________

3rd degree (including the anal sphincter) ___________________________

4th degree (including the tissue of the rectum) ___________________________

BLOOD LOSS ___________________________

DELIVERY OF PLACENTA
Spontaneous ___________________________

Manual Removal ___________________________

PLACENTAL PROBLEMS
Placenta abruptio ___________________________
(Placenta separates from the wall of the uterus before birth of the baby)

Placenta previa ___________________________
(Placenta is attached to the wall of the uterus at or near the cervix. Makes a Cesarean
birth necessary because the placenta would be delivered before the baby, cutting off the
baby's blood supply before birth.)

Retained placenta____
(Placenta does not separate from the wall of the uterus within a reasonable length of time after the birth of the baby, although the time considered "reasonable" varies with practitioner and institution. A normal placental separation can take as long as 20 to 30 minutes. Breast-feeding helps the placenta separate.)

Other

OTHER PROCEDURES
Dilatation and curettage (D & C)____
Other (specify and describe)   ____

SPECIAL DIAGNOSTIC TESTS IN LABOR

ELECTRONIC FETAL MONITORING

This is a procedure whereby the fetal heart rate (FHR) can be continually listened to and its rate recorded throughout labor. It can be done externally by means of two belts placed around the laboring woman's abdomen. One belt records the FHR, the other the uterine contractions. Both of these can also be monitored internally, with a small wire (electrode) placed onto the baby's scalp and a tube (catheter) placed into the uterus. Some practitioners use routine monitoring, although long-term effects of external monitoring are unknown. Short-term side effects of internal monitoring include possible scalp and uterine infection. The FHR in labor can be listened to with a fetoscope by an experienced practitioner and adequately assesssed in most women not at risk.

FETAL SCALP pH

If the FHR shows a pattern that indicates possible distress, a direct sample of the fetus's blood can be taken through the vagina from the baby's scalp. This sample is tested for pH—the acidity of the blood. pH gives an indication of the oxygen content of the baby's blood. Side effects include bleeding or infection at the site of the incision. A method of continuous monitoring of blood pH throughout labor is now being developed and tested.

BIRTH DIARY

Women have said that labor is the most difficult experience to live through and the easiest to forget. Though it may be fresh in your mind immediately afterward, it is amazing how easily memories can be dimmed by sleepless nights, bouts of baby's crying, and sore breasts or dirty bottles. Then, too, the joys of baby's first smile, first words, first steps—all his or her never-ending firsts—soon seem to overshadow what becomes the mere fact of birth.

Yet, how wonderful it would be to have a record of your feelings at seeing your baby for the first time, to remember always your first words, your first thoughts. You might also want to record the confusion, frustration, pain, fear, exhaustion—even anger—that you felt during labor and delivery, the effort of pushing, the exhilaration of birth. This part of women's lives has so long been considered taboo or actually missed during the years of heavily sedated labors that it has been largely lost to recent human history.

It is time for us to reclaim the birth experience as part of our lives. So, write whatever feelings you have; then, pass this page on to your labor partner, to your baby's father, to grandparents, or to anyone else with you at the birth or soon afterwards. You will be delighted to reread it in the future, to compare your feelings to other women's, and to share it someday with your child.

BIRTH DIARY

The experience of labor

Perceptions of the baby—first words and thoughts

THE POSTPARTUM PERIOD

Postpartum means after birth. It is defined as the period of six weeks immediately following delivery. This is the time considered necessary for a woman's internal organs to return as closely as they will to their nonpregnant condition.

Enormous changes occur in a woman's body as a result of delivery. Some practitioners call the first postpartum hour the "fourth stage of labor." A woman needs to be cared for closely at this time, to be watched for bleeding or other changes that might signal the need for medical intervention. Some hospitals actually have a "recovery room" for this significant hour. Of course, close supervision by a midwife, doctor, nurse, or other experienced birth attendant can be provided anywhere.

When the placenta separates from the uterus (womb), it leaves an open wound. The muscles of the uterus contract to apply pressure to this area, thus preventing excessive bleeding. The uterus must remain contracted. Usually this occurs naturally, especially if you breast-feed. Sometimes, medications need to be given to help this contraction. The uterus should be checked frequently during the immediate postpartum period. If it is contracted it feels like a hard, tight knot near the navel (umbilicus). Blood pressure, pulse, and respirations should also be monitored, to make sure that there is no hidden bleeding.

Each woman responds individually to the experience of birth. This response depends on the length and strength of her labor, her general state of health and nutrition, any medical and obstetrical problems, medications given, amount of blood lost, and the condition of the baby. It also varies with the emotional support received during labor and delivery and personal characteristics. It is difficult to predict whether you will want to get out of bed almost immediately or want nothing more than to sleep. Many women are hungry or thirsty right after birth. People often bring food and drink to the hospital or birth center during labor to eat after the baby is born. Some birth centers have kitchens so that the woman's partner can prepare her favorite dish—which you've both earned. Champagne is a favorite for postbirth celebrations.

If your newborn is healthy, you should have immediate access to him or her. Some practitioners put the baby on the mother's abdomen right at delivery. Partners sometimes cut the cord. There is no reason mothers and fathers or other partners cannot touch a newborn. There is no need for a newly delivered infant without problems to be placed in an incubator or isolette for warmth. Babies should be dried to avoid getting chilly. Studies have shown that babies placed in skin-to-skin contact with their mothers maintain their temperatures quite well.

Babies who are not medicated during labor are usually wide awake and alert for the first hour or so of their lives. This is a good time for them to get acquainted with their parents and to start the process of learning to nurse. Immediate nursing has benefits for the mother as well. It stimulates the release of the hormone oxytocin, nature's way of helping the uterus contract. This early meeting of parents and baby begins the "bonding" process. A number of hospitals—at the prodding of parents—encourage women to be awake during Cesarean births.

Partners are present for the birth, and bonding takes place as soon as the baby is checked by a pediatrician.

In the "Leboyer" method of gentle birth, babies are born into quiet, dimly lit rooms with soft music playing. The newborn is quickly placed into a warm bath, which provides a familiar environment. Pictures have shown these newborns smiling in their baths. If you are interested in this method, read the book by Dr. Leboyer listed at the end of this introduction. Decide which parts of the gentle birth process you would like for your baby and discuss them with your practitioner or those in your clinic. We like the concept of gentleness at birth, but prefer to give the baby to the parents to hold and cuddle.

Experiences during the postpartum period vary with place of delivery. We suggest that in choosing a practitioner or clinic for your prenatal care, you look into the policies of the setting where you will deliver. You will be most comfortable and happy at a place whose guidelines follow your own beliefs most closely. Use the "Birth Plan" (p. 193) to help you determine those areas about which you have preferences. Unfortunately, the amount of choice you have depends to a large extent on the part of the country in which you live and your economic resources.

Out-of-hospital birth centers encourage bonding and breast-feeding on demand and accept parental input for postpartum needs. Families generally stay in birth centers for twelve to twenty-four hours after delivery. In home births, of course, there are no fixed routines. Practitioners and parents should agree beforehand on how they want the postpartum period managed.

Hospital postpartum policies vary greatly. Postpartum stays are usually two to three days after birth, although many women prefer to leave earlier. After a Cesarean birth, hospital stays are generally five to seven days. Many hospitals provide "rooming-in" for mothers and babies. This allows for individual care of new babies by their own mothers. Rooming-in facilitates feeding when the baby is hungry. In some places, fathers can visit all day. They stay in the same room as mother and baby, holding and caring for baby as much as desired. Sister and brother (sibling) visiting hours may be provided. In other institutions, babies are kept in central nurseries and brought to mothers only for scheduled feedings, usually every four hours. Too often, fathers get to see their child only through glass.

Many parents object to the fact that hospital routines often don't take individual circumstances into consideration. In some institutions, for example, after a Cesarean birth the baby is kept in an isolette (incubator) for twelve to twenty-four hours for observation. This may be done regardless of the baby's condition or the parents' desire for rooming-in. Hospital policies often require that babies be kept in the nursery, away from their mothers, whenever the mother has a temperature of 100.4°F. This may be done even though low-grade fevers are often quite normal, especially within the first twenty-four hours after birth or if breasts are engorged. If you have a choice of hospitals in your community and your health does not require that you deliver in the hospital with the most advanced technology, you may wish to choose a practitioner or clinic associated with the most flexible institution or the one whose policies most closely reflect your own philosophy.

Most hospitals offer child-care classes on the postpartum floor. Parents can take advantage of the availability of experienced nurses to ask questions about topics such as bathing and feeding. Be careful, however. Not all hospital personnel will share your perspectives. You may be discouraged, for example, from breast-feeding by staff who don't understand that breast milk is digested more quickly than formula so breast-fed babies are hungry more often.

Physical and emotional changes occur rapidly during the postpartum weeks. Probably the most pervasive postpartum feeling is fatigue, which can make all adjustments seem even more difficult.

The body has many postpartum tasks to accomplish. The uterus must return to its nonpregnant size. At the same time, it must shed its lining. This is done through a vaginal discharge called lochia. Lochia feels similar to a menstrual period, which it is not. The amount of discharge, never more than a heavy period, should decrease with time. It should also change from red to pink to brown and finally become colorless. This occurs as the uterus returns to its nonpregnant state, a process called involution. Rest is needed for the uterus to involute without complications. This seems almost a biologic cruelty, since caring for a tiny baby is a job with little provision for rest. The help of friends and family can be invaluable during this time. When husbands or partners are actively involved, the postpartum period is made much easier.

The extra fluid that normally accumulates in the body during pregnancy is lost in the days following. You will perspire a lot and urinate frequently in the early postpartum period. This is natural and should not be a cause for concern. Make sure you drink a lot of water or juice.

The perineum needs time to heal if an episiotomy was done or if a laceration occurred during delivery. Warm water aids healing. It helps to keep the area clean. Always wipe yourself gently, from front to back.

See the section "Infant Feeding" on page 270 for information about breast-feeding. If you are not breast-feeding, your milk must dry up. Some practitioners prescribe medications to aid this process, but these are not without side effects. Letting nature do the job is usually somewhat uncomfortable for a day or two. The breasts will fill up in a few days after birth, causing tenderness and perhaps even a mild fever. Ice packs and a tightly fitting bra or binder help. Small doses of aspirin or acetaminophen (Tylenol) can be taken for the pain and fever.

Menstrual periods may return within six to eight weeks for bottle-feeding women but may take many months to return if you are breast-feeding. Ovulation—the release of the egg cell—can occur at any time twelve to sixteen days before your first period. Therefore, it is possible to become pregnant before menstruation begins.

Most couples want to know when they can have sex after a pregnancy. Some practitioners advise waiting for the four- to six-week postpartum checkup, recommending sexual contact other than intercourse until then. Some cultures specify a definite waiting period before sex can be resumed. Physically, however, as long as you are not bleeding heavily and there is no pain, sex is not at all dangerous. The length of time necessary for comfort during intercourse varies. It may be a week if you did not have stitches or three or four weeks if you had a large cut. Let your own body be your guide.

Once you begin having intercourse you must consider birth control. We recommend foam and condoms as the best postpartum contraceptive. A diaphragm cannot be used until involution is complete. Most practitioners wait until the first menstrual period to insert an IUD. Some will insert it at your four- or six-week postpartum check, if your uterus is involuted and you have not yet had sex. Many practitioners prescribe the pill immediately postpartum for non-breast-feeding women. Others advise waiting until your first menstrual period. This gives your body a chance to resume normal functioning. It also takes you past the danger period for developing postpartum blood clots, a danger increased with pill use. (See the section on "Contraceptive History," p. 140, for more information on birth-control methods.)

Use these postpartum charts to record physical changes. Be especially alert to any of the danger signs listed and contact your practitioner or clinic should they occur. Good nutrition is essential for all postpartum processes. See the section "Nutrition" for more information about dietary needs and use the nutrition charts in that section with care. Exercise is another must to restore muscle strength. Review the section "Exercise" and use the exercise chart provided to plan an effective exercise routine.

What Now? A Handbook for New Parents by Mary Lou Rozdilsky and Barbara Banet (New York, Charles Scribner's Sons, 1975) is an easy-to-read book on postpartum care for parents. It gives a lot of practical advice. We suggest reading *Parent-Infant Bonding* by Marshall Klaus and John Kennel (St. Louis, the C. V. Mosby Company, revised 1982) for a discussion about the value of early contact with infants. If you are interested in a Leboyer birth, the book to read is *Birth Without Violence* by Frederick Leboyer, (New York, Alfred A. Knopf, 1975). We feel compelled, however, to caution you about Dr. Leboyer's negative attitudes toward mothers.

IMMEDIATE POSTPARTUM PERIOD
("Fourth Stage of Labor"—Birth to 1 hour after birth)

MEDICATIONS GIVEN (See chart, pp. 218–220)

REASON	NAME	DOSAGE	INTRA-VENOUSLY	BY INJECTION (INTRAMUSCULARLY)	BY MOUTH (ORALLY)
			CHECK OFF HOW GIVEN		
To keep uterus contracted					
Other (specify) _______					

PROBLEMS IMMEDIATELY POSTPARTUM

PROBLEM	TREATMENT
Postpartum bleeding (hemorrhage)___________	
Other___________	

POSTPARTUM STAY IN HOSPITAL

Number of days in hospital___________________________

MEDICATIONS GIVEN (see chart, pp. 218–220)

REASON	NAME	DATE	DOSAGE	HOW GIVEN
To keep uterus contracted				
To dry up breast milk				
For pain relief				
Iron/vitamins				
For sleep				
To have a bowel movement				
RhoGAM (If Rh negative)				
Other___________				

LAB TESTS TAKEN	DATE	RESULT
Hematocrit		
Other___________		
Other___________		

COMPLICATIONS OR PROBLEMS (specify and describe):

____

____

BLOOD TRANSFUSION: Number of pints given___________

If reaction occurred, describe___________

SIX-WEEK POSTPARTUM PERIOD

MEDICATIONS GIVEN TO TAKE AT HOME					
			HOW TO TAKE		
TYPE OF MEDICATION/REASON	**NAME**	**DOSAGE**	**HOW OFTEN**	**WITH/ WITHOUT MEALS**	**SPECIAL INSTRUC- TIONS**
Iron/vitamins					
Other_____________					
Other_____________					

CONTRACEPTION TO USE AT HOME (See "Contraceptive History" for more information.)
Foam and Condoms_____________

Other_____________

RESUMPTION OF SEX
Pain?   Yes_____________   No_____________
Other problems_____________

POSTPARTUM DANGER SIGNS AND PROBLEMS

NOTIFY YOUR PRACTITIONER!		
SYMPTOM	**POSSIBLE PROBLEM**	**DATE**
Increased bleeding/clots	May be due to too much activity. If it does not sub- side with rest, may be a postpartum hemorrhage.	
Pain: Abdominal	May be a uterine infection.	
Vaginal	May be poorly healing episiotomy or hematoma. Some pain is expected but should decrease.	
Perineal	May be poorly healing episiotomy. Some pain is expected but should decrease.	
Rectal	May be hemorrhoids or poorly healing 3rd or 4th degree laceration.	
Leg pain	May be a sign of blood clot in the vein— thrombophlebitis.	
Reddened, swollen, warm, or hardened area on leg Or reddened streak along leg, may feel like a rope inside the leg	May be a sign of a blood clot in the vein— thrombophlebitis	
Pain with urination, urinary urgency and frequency	Urinary frequency alone is normal in the postpar- tum period. Pain on the outside area may be soreness due to episiotomy, lacerations, or abra- sions. Internal pain while urinating, along with urgency (a strong feeling that you must urinate) and frequency might be a sign of a urinary-tract in- fection, especially if you urinate only small amounts.	
Fever/Chills	If mild, may be breast engorgement, but can signify infection after the first 24 hours.	
Foul smelling discharge (lochia)	May be postpartum infection.	

TWO-WEEK POSTPARTUM PRACTITIONER VISIT AFTER A CESAREAN BIRTH

DATE________________________________

QUESTIONS TO ASK

____

____

____

FINDINGS   COMMENTS

Incision: Healing?___________   Not healing?________________________

Uterus: Involuting?___________   Not involuting?________________________

Blood pressure:_______________

Other_______________________

LABORATORY TESTS   RESULTS

Hematocrit________________________   ________________________

Other________________________   ________________________

MEDICATIONS GIVEN

MEDICATION	REASON	DOSAGE	SPECIAL INSTRUCTIONS

OTHER TREATMENTS________________________________

DATE OF NEXT VISIT________________________________

FOUR- TO SIX-WEEK POSTPARTUM PRACTITIONER VISIT

DATE_______________________________________

QUESTIONS TO ASK

____

____

____

FINDINGS

Breasts	Normal_________________________	Other_________________
Uterus	Involuted?______________________	Not involuted?__________
Perineum	Healing?_______________________	Not healing?___________
Vagina	Healed?____________ Not healed?________	Muscle tone________
Cesarean incision	Healing?_______________________	Not healed?____________

Blood pressure_______________________________

Other____

LABORATORY TESTS   RESULTS

Hematocrit_________   _________________

Pap test (if needed)   _________________

Other_________   _________________

MEDICATIONS GIVEN

MEDICATION	REASON	DOSAGE	SPECIAL INSTRUCTIONS

OTHER TREATMENTS GIVEN_________________________________

CONTRACEPTIVE GIVEN___________________________________
(Also record in section "Contraceptive History," p. 140)

POSTPARTUM DIARY

The emotional ups and downs of pregnancy do not end with birth. The entry of a newborn into a family always brings new feelings. Newborns are totally helpless little beings. Suddenly you are responsible for the complete care of another. Insecurity, fear, and doubt are natural emotional responses. So, too, are elation and joy. Sometimes these opposite feelings come and go at an alarming pace, leaving a fatigued new mother quite bewildered.

The "postpartum blues" has become a commonly seen phenomenon in our culture. It leaves new mothers weepy without knowing why, sad with no apparent reason. No one really knows how widespread this experience is. Many attribute it to rapid hormonal changes. Some people believe that postpartum blues increase as a result of hospital practices that distance women from their birth experiences. These include heavily medicated labors and deliveries, lack of emotional support during birth, and separation of mothers and babies.

Sometimes you may have ambivalent feelings toward your baby. These are understandable. There you are, still tired from labor and birth, perhaps with a sore bottom and/or belly, learning a brand-new job, wondering how you will make it through each day. Relationships between partners change as the family expands to include a child. Old patterns of relating may need adjustment. Sexual needs may change, at least temporarily.

Single parents have different adjustments to make. You may live with other family members and their relationship to your new baby must be worked out. Women living alone will have to arrange for help during the early weeks. If you need or want to return to work soon—whether you are single or not—caretaking arrangements have to be made. Both financial and emotional considerations become vital.

If your newborn has any problems at all, your postpartum feelings will be affected. You will be extra fatigued if your baby requires prolonged hospitalization and you must visit daily. Depression, anxiety, and fear are expected. In this case, it is especially valuable to voice and share these feelings.

Give yourself this diary as a gift. Take a few minutes from time to time to be alone, to absorb and understand your new experiences with your child. As she or he grows, you can reread and remember these first weeks. You will appreciate your growth as a parent.

POSTPARTUM DIARY

1st week

2nd week

3rd week

4th week

5th week

6th week

COMMONLY USED MEDICATIONS IN CHILDBEARING

An area of ongoing debate in medicine today concerns the use of medications. This presents a great dilemma for people with health problems, as it does for practitioners. Questions arise concerning when to medicate, what drug to use and whether to use drugs for prevention (prophylaxis). Some practitioners tend to be aggressive or interventionist in relation to their use of drugs; others are more cautious, more inclined to give nature a chance before intervening.

Practitioners rely on analyses of risks versus benefits when prescribing drugs. Unfortunately, benefits are often more obvious and immediate than risks, easier to evaluate and given more attention in drug advertisements. It is a perhaps shocking truth that practitioners get most of their information about drugs from literature prepared by drug companies or from drug-company "detail" persons. Detail persons are essentially salespersons.

This section provides a list of some common drugs used during times when we are vulnerable—pregnancy, labor and delivery, and the postpartum period. A list of commonly used drugs in childhood can be found on page 296, near the end of the section "Childhood Practitioner Visits." The inclusion of these sections in this book is *not* an endorsement of the use of any of these products. Its purpose is to acquaint you with names of drugs, their uses, benefits, and possible side effects to help you be a more informed consumer and to facilitate your record-keeping. We have included chemical (or generic) names as well as common brand names of various drugs. Since many drugs are produced by a number of different companies, we may not have included *all* brand names for each. The inclusion of one brand name over another in no way endorses that product over the same product produced by another company. Indeed, we support the concept of prescribing by generic name so that less expensive versions of the same drug can be purchased.

Since prescription writing is considered a confidential act of a physician, little information is available on specific rates of prescribing specific drugs. For this reason, the actual drug names included may not represent the most widely used products in all cases. Some of the material for the pregnancy and childhood sections is based on data supplied by the National Disease and Therapeutic Index, which showed categories of the most commonly used drugs in prenatal care and among children up to the age of five. The data supplied are copyrighted by IMS America, Ltd., and have been used with permission. No material has been reprinted as supplied. Another useful source for the section on drugs in labor and delivery was The March of Dimes Birth Defects Foundation module, *Selected Drugs Used During Labor and Delivery: Effects on the Fetus and Neonate* by Jane Pohodich, R.N., M.N., (March of Dimes, New York, 1980).

SOME COMMONLY USED MEDICATIONS IN PREGNANCY

TYPE OF DRUG	CHEMICAL (GENERIC) NAME	EXAMPLES OF BRAND NAME	HOW GIVEN/ USUAL DOSAGE
PRENATAL VITAMINS	Usually contain multi-vitamins and various minerals: Vitamins A, B Complex, C, D, and E; Iron, Magnesium, Calcium, Phosphorus, Zinc, Copper, Iodine; Exact composition varies with specific vitamin.	Natalins Pramilet Stuart Prenatal Filibon Others	By mouth One tablet once a day
IRON	Ferrous gluconate Ferrous sulfate Ferrous fumarate	Fergon Feosol Mol-Iron Ferro-Sequels (also contains dioctyl sodium sulfosuccinate) (see below)	By mouth One tablet one, two or three times a day
TO PREVENT NAUSEA	Combination of: Doxylamine succinate and Pyridoxine hydrochloride (Vitamin B_6)	Bendectin	By mouth Two tablets at bedtime; 1 in the morning and afternoon if needed (We do not advise using this drug.)
TO SOFTEN STOOL	Dioctyl sodium sulfosuccinate	Colace	By mouth 50–300 mgs/day usually given three times a day
LAXATIVES—TO STIMULATE BOWEL MOVEMENTS	Dioctyl sodium sulfosuccinate with casanthranol Psyllium hydrophilic mucilloid (made from grain)	Peri-Colace Metamucil Many others	By mouth One or two capsules or tablespoons at bedtime By mouth One teaspoonful 1–3 times/day
ANTACIDS	Aluminum Hydroxide, Magnesium, and Simethicone Aluminum Hydroxide and Magnesium	Mylanta Maalox Gelusil	By mouth One or two tablets or teaspoonsful between meals or at bedtime

POSSIBLE SIDE EFFECTS	COMMENTS
Can overdose on fat-soluble vitamins—A, D, E. (Do not take more than prescribed amount of medication.)	May take additional supplements as needed. Examples are: Vitamin B_6 for nausea; Calcium if you can't drink milk or eat milk products; Vitamin B_{12} if you eat no animal products; Folic acid for some types of anemia; Vitamin C to possibly aid the body's use of iron and folic acid. Many practitioners give vitamins routinely but they are most likely unnecessary if your diet is adequate. We recommend *no* medication—even vitamins—in the first 12 weeks (first trimester) of pregnancy.
Stomach upsets; Nausea and vomiting; Constipation	Take with meals to reduce stomach upsets. Do not take with milk or milk products which interfere with the body's use of iron. Many practitioners give iron routinely but it is unnecessary if the iron in your blood is good. If your hemoglobin and hematocrit remain within normal limits through pregnancy, they are not necessary.
Has been implicated in two studies in causing birth defects.	Is currently under investigation to determine its role in possible teratogenesis. Dry crackers and other carbohydrates (such as popcorn) and carbonated beverages can alleviate nausea and vomiting. Keep at your bedside and eat before arising. Eat small, frequent meals. Avoid fatty, fried foods. The nausea and vomiting of early pregnancy are generally not serious and subside with time.
No known effects on fetus.	Often given because of the constipation caused by taking iron and problems with hemorrhoids so common in pregnancy.
Laxatives can be habit-forming and can cause excessive excretion of important body chemicals.	To avoid constipation, eat an increased amount of fiber (whole grains, fresh fruits and vegetables). Prune juice is a good natural laxative. Drink lots of fluid and make sure you go when you feel the urge! Exercise.
May interfere with body's ability to use iron. (Do not overuse.)	To reduce gas, avoid gas-forming foods such as beans, cabbage, radishes. Avoid fatty or fried foods. Drink liquids between meals. To avoid heartburn, do not lie down immediately after eating.

SOME COMMONLY USED MEDICATIONS IN LABOR ONLY

TYPE OF DRUG	CHEMICAL (GENERIC) NAME	EXAMPLES OF BRAND NAME	HOW GIVEN/ USUAL DOSAGE
HORMONE: TO INDUCE OR STIMULATE LABOR	Oxytocin	Pitocin Syntocinon	By mouth (buccal; given under the tongue) or Intravenous (IV), mixed with fluids (saline or electrolyte solution). Start with small dose and gradually increase.
FOR SLEEP IN EARLY LABOR	Secobarbital Pentobarbital	Seconal Nembutal	By mouth 100 mg (1 tablet) at night.
FOR PAIN RELIEF: ANALGESIA (REDUCTION OF PAIN) NARCOTICS	Meperidine Alphaprodine	Demerol Nisentil	Intramuscular (IM injection) or IV 25–100 mg no more than every 3 to 4 hours. Subcutaneous (shallow injection, under the skin) 40–60 mg no more than every 2 hours
ANESTHESIA (COMPLETE PAIN RELIEF)	Paracervical block uses form of local anesthetic, for example, Lidocaine Mepivacaine Bupivacaine	Xylocaine Carbocaine Marcaine	Through the vagina, injected around the cervix. .25–1% solution used, approx. 10 cc given
FOR RELAXATION: TRANQUILIZERS GIVEN TO AID RELAXATION OR TO INCREASE EFFECT OF NARCOTIC	Diazepam Hydroxyzine Promazine Promethazine	Valium Vistaril Sparine Phenergan	5–10 mg IV or IM 25–100 mg, IM 25–50 mgs IV or IM

POSSIBLE SIDE EFFECTS			
TO MOTHER	ON LABOR	TO BABY	COMMENTS
Water intoxication, if too much water is given; can lead to convulsions.	Tetanic contractions: contractions that are too long or too strong.	Fetal Distress. Some studies have shown higher rates of hyper-bilirubinemia in newborns after labor inductions (See "Problems of the Newborn," p. 258)	Not to be given if mother has shown previous sensitivity. Not to be given if mother has had previous uterine surgery or if pelvis is too small for size of baby. The FDA has prohibited the use of oxytocin for elective inductions of labor; there must be a medical reason for its use. Labor cannot be induced for convenience of physician or mother because of risk of prematurity.
Drowsiness, fatigue.	May slow labor.	Central-nervous-system depression. Long-term effects unknown.	*Never* to be taken with alcohol. Not to be given in active labor, especially near the time of birth.
Nausea, vomiting, drowsiness, disorientation, respiratory depression (especially in large doses).	May slow labor.	Central-nervous-system depression. Can depress baby's breathing at birth if given too near to birth. Long-term effects unknown but drugs have been found in baby's urine days after birth.	Demerol is not to be given IV one to two hours before birth or IM two to three hours before birth. Nisentil is not to be given one hour before birth. Naloxone (Narcan) can be given to baby as an injection after birth to counteract the effects of narcotics if baby is having breathing difficulties at birth from the effects of the drugs.
Rare, unless sensitive to drug.	May depress uterine contractions, slowing labor.	May cause a drop in fetal heart rate, usually short-term. May cause depressed breathing at birth if given 30 mins. before.	Because of possible effect on fetal heart rate, baby's heart must be carefully monitored following a paracervical block. Provides very short-term pain relief, approx. 1 hour.
Dizziness, decreased blood pressure, drowsiness, disorientation. In the presence of severe pain, may cause increased anxiety rather than relaxation.		Central-nervous-system depression. Difficulty breathing if given close to birth. Long-term effects unknown but drugs can remain active for days after birth.	Effects cannot be counteracted after birth with any other medications.

SOME COMMONLY USED MEDICATIONS IN LABOR AND/OR DELIVERY

TYPE OF DRUG	CHEMICAL (GENERIC) NAME	EXAMPLES OF BRAND NAMES	HOW GIVEN/ USUAL DOSAGE
EPIDURAL: FOR ANESTHESIA (pain relief)	Epidural anesthesia uses form of anesthetic agent, for example, Chloroprocaine Bupivacaine	Nesacaine Marcaine	Injected into the "epidural" space in the spinal canal, below the level of the spinal cord. May be given as single dose or, in labor, through a tube placed in the canal so dose can be repeated.

SOME COMMONLY USED MEDICATIONS IN DELIVERY ONLY

LOCAL ANESTHESIA: FOR CUTTING AND/OR REPAIR OF EPISIOTOMY	Lidocaine	Xylocaine	Injected into the perineum, the area where episiotomy is cut. 1% solution used; approx. 10 cc.
PUDENDAL: FOR CUTTING AND/OR REPAIR OF EPISIOTOMY	Lidocaine	Xylocaine	Injected through the vagina to block the pudendal nerve, which causes anesthesia in the perineal area.
SADDLE BLOCK: FOR ANESTHESIA OF THE AREA OF BODY THAT WOULD TOUCH A SADDLE IF YOU WERE RIDING.	For example: Tetracaine	Pontocaine	Injected into the spinal canal at level necessary for anesthesia.
SPINAL: ANESTHESIA FOR AREA BELOW THE BREASTS.	See above		
GENERAL ANESTHESIA: TO PUT YOU TO SLEEP.	Many agents For example: Thiopental May be given with nitrous oxide gas.	Pentothal	Given IV Gas given through facial mask or nose clip.

POSSIBLE SIDE EFFECTS			
TO MOTHER	**ON LABOR**	**TO BABY**	**COMMENTS**
Decreased blood pressure. Should not cause headache if done properly, but if done improperly, may cause headache.	May slow labor. May decrease the ability to push and thus increase the possibility of forceps delivery.	May cause fetal distress if decrease in mother's blood pressure persists. Long-term effects on baby unknown, but some central-nervous-system effects are suspected.	Should not be given to woman who has shown previous sensitivity to drug used.

TO MOTHER	ON LABOR	TO BABY	COMMENTS
Allergic reactions. Respiratory and cardiac problems if inadvertently injected into a blood vessel.	Usually none because given just before delivery or postpartum just for repair. Pudendal may make pushing more difficult.	None if given after birth. Usually none if given just before delivery, but can depress baby if absorbed quickly or given into a blood vessel.	Should not be given to woman who has shown previous sensitivity. If allergic to anesthetic given by dentist, tell your practitioner. With proper technique, should not be injected into blood vessel.
Sometimes, spinal headache.	None if given just before delivery.	Should not affect baby if given just before delivery.	Used for delivery only with forceps.
Spinal headache. Decreased blood pressure. Respiratory depression. Bladder dysfunction.	See above		Used for delivery by Cesarean section only.
Respiratory depression. Postanesthesia blood clots, pneumonia.	None if given just before delivery.	Respiratory depression.	Used for forceps delivery or Cesarean section. Must have a tube in the nose or mouth during general anesthesia to prevent breathing of any vomited material.

SOME COMMONLY USED MEDICATIONS IN THE POSTPARTUM PERIOD

TYPE OF DRUG	CHEMICAL (GENERIC) NAME	EXAMPLES OF BRAND NAME	HOW GIVEN/ USUAL DOSAGE
TO KEEP UTERUS CON- TRACTED AND PREVENT POSTPARTUM BLEEDING.	Oxytocin	Pitocin Syntocinon	IM (intramuscular injec- tion), 5–10 units. IV (intravenous), 5–20 units in 500–1000 cc of fluid. Usually given imme- diately postpartum.
	Ergonovine Methylergonovine	Ergotrate Methergine	IM or by mouth, 0.2 mg every 6–12 hours for 2 days. Same as above, given every 4 hours for 2 days.
TO DRY UP BREAST MILK IF FORMULA FEEDING.	Bromocriptine Testosterone and Estradiol	Parlodel Deladumone OB	By mouth 2.5 mg for 14 days with meals. IM, just after birth, 2 cc.
FOR PAIN RELIEF	Acetaminophen	Tylenol	By mouth, 1 or 2 tabs, 3–4 times a day. (325 mg per tablet)
	Codeine		By mouth, 7.5–60 mg every four hours.

POSSIBLE SIDE EFFECTS	COMMENTS
Increased cramplike pains.	Many practitioners routinely give oxytocin postpartum to prevent postpartum bleeding. It is generally considered safe for postpartum use at the levels given, although it is not always necessary, especially for breast-feeding women.
Increased blood pressure. Nausea and vomiting. Increased cramplike pains.	Not to be given to woman with elevated blood pressure. Not to be given to woman who has shown previous sensitivity.
Decreased blood pressure. Nausea and vomiting. Dizziness. Fatigue. Occasional fainting, cramping, diarrhea. Blood clots. Voice changes (deepening). Increased hair growth.	Not to be given to woman sensitive to any "ergot" preparation. Sometimes, breast fullness (engorgement) occurs when medication is stopped. Not to be given to woman with breast or genital cancer or to woman with a history of thrombophlebitis or any blood clots. Estrogen has been shown to be teratogenic when given during pregnancy. Long-term effects of postpartum use unknown. If no medication is taken to dry up breast milk, bottle-feeding women can use these remedies for relief of discomfort: ice packs, a supportive bra or binder, and mild analgesic such as acetaminophen.
Rare, but can damage the liver with overdosage.	Should not be given to a woman with previous sensitivity.
May be habit-forming. May cause drowsiness. May cause sleepiness in baby if taken by breast-feeding woman.	May be given with Tylenol for increased pain relief. Best to take after breast-feeding.

SOME COMMONLY USED MEDICATIONS IN THE POSTPARTUM PERIOD (continued)

TYPE OF DRUG	CHEMICAL (GENERIC) NAME	EXAMPLES OF BRAND NAME	HOW GIVEN/ USUAL DOSAGE
IRON AND VITAMINS	See "Pregnancy" section for information		
FOR SLEEPING	Flurazepam	Dalmane	By mouth, 15–30 mg, at bedtime.
	Secobarbital	Seconal	By mouth, 100 mg, at bedtime.
	Pentobarbital	Nembutal	
TO HAVE BOWEL MOVEMENT	Milk of Magnesia (MOM)		By mouth, 2 Tbs. or 30 ccs at night.
LAXATIVES:	Dioctyl sodium sulfosuccinate with casanthranol	Peri-Colace Dialose Plus	1–2 capsules at bedtime.
ENEMAS:	Soap suds enema Mineral oil	Fleets	Rectally
TO SOFTEN STOOL:	Dioctyl sodium sulfosuccinate	Colace Dialose	By mouth, 50–300 mg daily, usually given 3 times a day.
TO PREVENT Rh SENSITIZATION	Rh_o (D) immune globulin	RhoGAM	IM, 1 vial within 72 hours after delivery.

SOME COMMONLY USED DRUGS IN THE NORMAL NEWBORN

TYPE OF DRUG	CHEMICAL (GENERIC) NAME	EXAMPLES OF BRAND NAME	HOW GIVEN/ USUAL DOSAGE
TO PREVENT OPHTHALMIA NEONATORUM CAUSED BY GONORRHEA	Silver nitrate ($AgNO_3$)		Eye drops.
	Tetracycline Erythromycin		Ointment to eye.
TO PREVENT BLEEDING	Vitamin K	AquaMephyton	IM 0.5–1 mg

POSSIBLE SIDE EFFECTS	COMMENTS
Dizziness, drowsiness. Habit-forming. Decreased blood pressure, respiratory depression. Rash if allergic. May cause drowsiness in baby if taken by breast-feeding woman.	Considered to give a more physiologic sleep than other sleeping pills. Changes normal sleep patterns so that fatigue may actually be increased with continued use. No sleeping pill should be given to woman with previous sensitivity or kidney, heart, or lung problems. *Never* use sleeping pills with alcohol.
Can lead to dependence. Injury to the bowel.	Laxatives and enemas are not to be used with nausea and vomiting or abdominal pain. Many postpartum women don't have a B.M. for quite a few days. This is normal since the digestive system slows down during labor and delivery and you usually eat little. It isn't necessary to have a B.M. soon after delivery if you are not uncomfortable. Eat whole grains, fresh fruits and vegetables and drink lots of water as natural aids to bowel function. Exercise.
Generally considered safe.	Should be given to a woman who has had a 3rd or 4th degree laceration (see section "Labor and Delivery," p. 189).

SEE "SPECIAL DIAGNOSTIC TESTS IN PREGNANCY," p. 176, FOR INFORMATION.

Baby will close eyes. Prevents eye contact with parents and environment. Inflammation for a few days after birth.	Required by law in almost all states. Other antibiotic ointments are sometimes used.
Pain and swelling at site of infection. Increased incidence of hyperbilirubinemia after Vitamin K is given.	See "The Newborn," p. 252, for more information.

NOTES

NOTES

The Second Experience

PREGNANCY (II)

Just as every child is different, every pregnancy is different. The majority of pregnancies are normal and uncomplicated, whether first, second, or after many children. Sometimes, however, a woman who had an easy, placid experience of the first pregnancy will be dismayed to find herself subjected to many pressures, or discomfort from nausea or headaches, the second time around. This also may work in reverse. It's possible for a woman who had a difficult pregnancy to dream of the perfect, golden experience she wished for—and to superimpose this dream over the expectations of her second pregnancy.

Variation of experience is normal and can even be expected. However, if common sense tells you that by comparing subsequent pregnancies with the first one you have cause for concern on some point, you should bring it to the attention of your practitioner or the practitioners in your clinic.

We have not repeated the Birth Plan or Birth Plan for Unexpected Situations for the second pregnancy. We refer you back to your first experience to see what choices you made then. Think about your labor and birth and remember what you actually did choose. Then decide if your plan will remain the same or change. You can use the same form for this pregnancy plan.

HEALTH DATA AT TIME OF CONCEPTION

MOTHER

Age_______________ Weight_______________ Height_______________

Occupation: Title_______________ Employer_______________ Department_______________

ILLNESS(ES)

At time of conception____

Recent exposure to infection: Date_______________ Specify nature_______________

MEDICATIONS TAKEN: Name_______________ Date(s)_______________
Other drug use____
Alcohol:

Type	# days per week used	# glasses per day
Beer		
Wine		
Hard Liquor		

Tobacco:

	# per day
Cigarettes	
Cigars	
Pipe	

Caffeine:

	# ounces or glasses per day
Colas and other sodas	
Coffee	
Tea	
Chocolate	

Pica (Unusual food cravings or ingestion of clay, dirt, ice, or laundry starch) Specify frequency and amount____

____

Date of conception, if known____

Last menstrual period: Date of first day_______________ Number of days_______________
     Amount of flow (normal/less than normal)_______________

Previous menstrual period____

Last contraceptive used: Type_______________ Date Discontinued_______________

Your calculation of your **E**stimated **D**ate of **C**onfinement (EDC) due date
     Subtract three months from the date of your last normal menstrual period and add seven days
     to the first day:____

See Medical, Obstetrical, and Family History for other relevant data.

HEALTH DATA AT TIME OF CONCEPTION

FATHER

Age______________ Weight______________ Height______________

Blood type and Rh______________

Occupation:

Title______________ Employer______________ Department______________

ILLNESS(ES)

At time of conception______________

Recent exposure to infection: Date______________ Specify nature______________

MEDICATIONS TAKEN:

Name______________ Date(s)______________

Other drug use______________

Alcohol:

Type	# days per week used	# glasses per day
Beer		
Wine		
Hard Liquor		

Tobacco:	# per day
Cigarettes	
Cigars	
Pipe	

Caffeine:	# ounces or glasses per day
Colas and other sodas	
Coffee	
Tea	
Chocolate	

Health of previous children (if any)______________

See Medical, Obstetrical, and Family History for other relevant data.

RECORD OF EXPOSURES DURING PREGNANCY

List all drugs taken.
Include prescription drugs, over-the-counter drugs, legal and illegal drugs.
Include tobacco, alcohol, and caffeine.
Include even those medications that seem harmless to you, like vitamins and cold pills, aspirin, or indigestion remedies.

NAME OF DRUG	DOSAGE	REASON TAKEN	DATES TAKEN	REACTIONS

RECORD OF EXPOSURES DURING PREGNANCY

List any chemical exposures, including occupational and environmental exposures.

CHEMICAL NAME	DATE(S)	LOCATION	EXPLANATION

List all X rays, including those taken by anyone other than your prenatal practitioner or clinic. Before any X ray is taken, make sure the practitioner is informed that you are pregnant. Include dental X rays.

DATE	PART OF BODY X-RAYED	HOSPITAL OR OFFICE	PRACTITIONER	REASON

ROUTINE PRENATAL LABORATORY TESTS
(See pp. 172 to 176 for explanations.)

TEST	DATE	RESULT
Pregnancy test (urine or blood)		
Pap smear		
Gonorrhea test		
Syphilis test (VDRL, ART, or Wasserman)		
Blood type		
Rh factor		
If negative, partner's Rh factor		
Complete blood count hemoglobin		
hematocrit		
Rubella immunity screen		

Sickle screen (if appropriate: See Family History)
   If positive:
   hemoglobin electrophoresis		

Partner's sickle screen		
Partner's hemoglobin electrophoresis		
Diabetic screening test (Fasting blood sugar and/or 2-hour postprandial)		
Urinalysis		
TB Skin Test (Tine or PPD)		

SPECIAL PRENATAL LABORATORY TESTS
(See pp. 176 to 179 for explanations.)

TEST	DATES	REASON	RESULT
Chest X ray			
Sonogram (Ultrasound)			
Amniocentesis			
Glucose tolerance test (GTT)			
Rh antibody screen (If Rh negative)			
Urine Culture and Sensitivity (C & S)			
Anemia work-up			

Viral studies
   TORCH: *T*oxoplasmosis, *R*ubella,
   *C*ytomegalovirus, *H*erpes			

Nonstress test (NST) or fetal activity test (FAT)			
Oxytocin challenge test (OCT)			
Amnioscopy			
Other (specify)_____________			

PRENATAL CARE PRACTITIONER VISITS

FIRST VISIT: Note any abnormalities on physical examination:

____

Results of clinical pelvimetry (size of pelvis):

Adequate_____________ Borderline____________ Contracted___________

MONTH/WEEK (*Fill in week**)	DATE	WEIGHT	BLOOD PRESSURE	URIN- ALYSIS: GLUCOSE/ PROTEIN	SIZE/ HEIGHT OF UTERUS
2nd month _______wk					
3rd month _______wk					
4th month _______wk					
5th month _______wk					______cms
6th month _______wk					______cms
7th month _______wk					______cms
_______wk					______cms
8th month _______wk					______cms
_______wk					______cms
9th month _______wk					______cms
_______wk					______cms
_______wk					______cms
_______wk					______cms
_______wk					______cms
_______wk					______cms
_______wk					______cms

* Practitioners calculate how pregnant you are in number of weeks. Your due date is forty weeks from the first day of your last period. At each visit, ask your practitioner how many weeks you are and fill in this information.

PRENATAL CARE PRACTITIONER VISITS

DATES TO RECORD: Practitioner's Calculation of your Estimated Date of Confinement (Due Date)____

Date of Quickening: The baby's first perceived movements. (It feels like a flutter.)____

Suggested schedule of visits for normal pregnancy: every 4 weeks to 6 months (24 wks.); every 3 weeks to 8 months (32 wks.); every other week to nine months (36 wks.); then every week.

FETAL HEART RATE (FHR) (*Specify fetoscope or doptone*)	POSITION OF FETUS	QUESTIONS FOR PRACTITIONER PROBLEMS NOTED OR INSTRUCTIONS PROCEDURES AND TREATMENTS

COMMON COMPLAINTS OR DISCOMFORTS OF PREGNANCY

Discuss relief measures with your practitioner or childbirth educator. Many home remedies that family members or friends can recommend work quite well. However: *don't use medication without discussing it first with your practitioner and don't reduce your dietary intake of any nutrient, including salt.*

DISCOMFORT	DATE(S) NOTED
Nausea and vomiting (early in pregnancy)	
Heartburn	
Breast tenderness	
Groin ache (round ligament pain)	
Leg pains or cramps	
Feet or ankle swelling	
Vaginal discharge (note color, odor, consistency, presence or absence of itch)	
Backaches (upper, mid, lower)_____________	
Hemorrhoids	
Constipation	
Varicose veins	
Dizziness	
Nasal congestion or nosebleeds	
Painful intercourse	
Mask of pregnancy (chloasma, facial skin discoloration)	
Tingling, numbness of fingers, arms	
Shortness of breath (late in pregnancy)	

RELIEF MEASURES TAKEN

COMPLICATIONS AND POSSIBLE SIGNS OF DANGER

SYMPTOM	POSSIBLE MEANING
BLEEDING: Amount______________ Color (pink, red, brown)______________ Consistency (thick, thin, clotted, possible tissue)______________ Associated activities (sex, orgasm, activity, vaginal exam)______________	Bleeding may be caused simply by cervical irritation. In early pregnancy, it may signal a possible miscarriage. Later in pregnancy, it may be due to placental separation from the uterus (abruptio) or to a placenta that is near the cervix (previa). Both are obstetrical emergencies.
CRAMPING	In early pregnancy, may be a sign of impending miscarriage. Later it may be premature labor, practice labor, or a symptom of a urinary tract or vaginal infection.
FEVER	A sign of infection—can itself cause premature labor.
HEADACHES: severe, prolonged BLURRY VISION CHEST PAIN SWELLING: especially face and hands	All of these may be signs of toxemia, a serious disease of pregnancy which can cause convulsions if not treated.
BAG OF WATER BREAKING (leakage of fluid—indicate color: clear, yellow, or brown) ______________	May increase both mother's and baby's chance of developing an infection. Yellow or brown fluid indicates the presence of meconium, which can mean fetal distress (except in a breech).
PAIN, URGENCY, OR FREQUENCY ON URINATION	A sign of a bladder or kidney infection, which can lead to premature labor.
EXCESSIVE VOMITING	Can lead to weight loss, dehydration, and "intrauterine growth retardation" (IUGR).
LEG PAINS	Can be thrombophlebitis, a blood clot.
DECREASED FETAL MOVEMENTS FELT (Near end of pregnancy)	A clear change in baby's movement pattern—may indicate baby is having a problem or it can simply be "lightening," the baby's moving down to become "fixed" in the pelvis.

DATE(S) NOTED	DATE PRACTITIONER CONTACTED	DIAGNOSIS AND TREATMENT (IF ANY)

PREGNANCY DIARY (II)

Emotionally as well as physically, there is wide variation between different pregnancies. Some worries may have diminished while others increase in importance. Sometimes financial pressure can be a greater source of concern as a family faces the expenses of a second child and perhaps a second loss of the mother's income, even if only temporarily.

One of the most common fears in a second pregnancy is that it will not be possible to love a second child as deeply as the first. It doesn't help when we are told, "Don't worry, it will all work out in the end." Sometimes, though, it is comforting to talk to other mothers who experienced this same misgiving and found relief with the birth and development of the second, unique, well-loved baby.

This diary for the second pregnancy is not intended to provide strict comparison with the first. Rather, it is to allow us to take each as the separate experience it must be.

PREGNANCY DIARY (II)

Second Month

Third Month

Fourth Month

Fifth Month

Sixth Month

Seventh Month

Eighth Month

Ninth Month

LABOR AND DELIVERY (II)

The general rule, as most women have heard, is for second and subsequent labors to be shorter and easier than the first. There are exceptions to this rule, as in the case of some women who had a first Cesarean birth and never dilated completely. Complications in a second labor may also mean a change in the expectation of a swifter second birth.

As in pregnancy and child rearing, it is best to approach each birth as a unique experience.

RECORD OF LABOR

Due Date____________________   Support Person(s)____________________

Date of Labor____________________   Number of weeks pregnant____________________

LENGTH OF LABOR

First stage (dilatation)   ____________________

Second stage (pushing)   ____________________

Third stage (placental)   ____________________

MEDICATIONS USED (See chart of Commonly Used Medications in Labor, pp. 214–216)

REASON	MEDICATION	DOSAGE/ NO. TIMES GIVEN	HOW GIVEN (BY MOUTH, INTRAVENOUSLY, BY INJECTION)
For induction of labor			
For stimulation of labor			
For sleep in early labor			
For pain relief (analgesia)			
For relaxation			
For episiotomy repair			
For medical or obstetrical problem(s) (Specify problem[s])__________			
For anesthesia			
If premature, medications used to stop labor			
If premature, medications given to mature baby's lungs			
Other (specify)			

If labor was induced or stimulated, give reason________________________________

If other medications were given, give reason__________________________________

Was electronic fetal monitor used? (Specify brand name of machine used.)__________
  Reason____
    Internal: For fetal heart rate   _______________________
                  For uterine contractions   _______________________
    External: For fetal heart rate   _______________________
                  For uterine contractions   _______________________
Was blood sample taken from baby?__________
Was scalp pH done?________________   Number of times____________
Reasons___________________________   Results__________________

X RAYS
How many were taken?______________________________________
Reasons: 1. to assess size of pelvis (pelvimetry)____________________
           2. to assess position of baby________________________
           3. other (specify)_________________________________

BAG OF WATERS
  Did bag of waters break spontaneously, or was it broken by obstetrician or
  midwife?____
  Before labor?________________   During labor?________________
  Color of fluid?________________   Specify number of cms:________
  Meconium?________________

COMPLICATIONS OF LABOR—SPECIFY AND DESCRIBE

RECORD OF DELIVERY

TYPE OF DELIVERY
  Normal spontaneous vaginal (NSVD)   ___________________________

  Forceps (specify low or mid)   ___________________________

  Vacuum   ___________________________

  Cesarean section (specify classical or transverse)   ___________________________

  Breech (specify spontaneous, assisted, breech
  extraction)   ___________________________

ANESTHESIA USED
  Specify type (see chart, p. 216)   ___________________________

PERINEUM
  Was episiotomy done?   ___________________________

    Type: Median   ___________________________

          Mediolateral (left or right)   ___________________________

  Laceration:
  1st degree (involving skin only or vaginal tissue)   ___________________________

  2nd degree (involving muscle)   ___________________________

  3rd degree (including the anal sphincter)   ___________________________

  4th degree (including the tissue of the rectum)   ___________________________

BLOOD LOSS   ___________________________

DELIVERY OF PLACENTA
Spontaneous ____

Manual Removal ____

PLACENTAL PROBLEMS
Placenta abruptio ____
(Placenta separates from the wall of the uterus before birth of the baby)

Placenta previa ____
(Placenta is attached to the wall of the uterus at or near the cervix. Makes a Cesarean birth necessary because the placenta would be delivered before the baby, cutting off the baby's blood supply before birth.)

Retained placenta ____
(Placenta does not separate from the wall of the uterus within a reasonable length of the time after the birth of the baby, although the time considered "reasonable" varies with practitioner and institution. A normal placental separation can take as long as 20 to 30 minutes. Breast-feeding helps the placenta separate.)

Other

OTHER PROCEDURES
Dilatation and curettage (D & C) ____
Other (specify and describe)   ____

BIRTH DIARY (II)

The experience of labor

Perceptions of the baby—first words and thoughts

THE POSTPARTUM PERIOD (II)

The postpartum period following a second delivery is generally easier than the first. The uterus has to work a bit harder to return to its normal size, so cramplike "afterpains" may be stronger, but otherwise the experience of having done it once makes adjustments less overwhelming.

Of course, each child is different. Your first may have slept through the night; your second may wake up every few hours. Your first may have had feeding difficulties; this child may eat peacefully and sleep contentedly afterward. You must always be prepared for the unexpected during the postpartum weeks.

A big difference is that a third family member needs to adjust along with the parents. "Sibling rivalry" is quite common, although its intensity depends on the first child's age. Most experts agree that the best way for parents to deal with jealous feelings is to accept them, to involve the older child in the care of the new baby, and to try to spend time alone with the older child whenever possible.

Use these postpartum charts to record physical and emotional changes. You may also want to use the postpartum diary this time to record the reactions of your firstborn.

IMMEDIATE POSTPARTUM PERIOD
("Fourth Stage of Labor"—Birth to 1 hour after birth)

MEDICATIONS GIVEN (See chart, pp. 218–220)

REASON	NAME	DOSAGE	CHECK OFF HOW GIVEN		
			INTRA-VENOUSLY	BY INJECTION (INTRAMUSCULARLY)	BY MOUTH (ORALLY)
To keep uterus contracted					
Other (specify) ___________					

PROBLEMS IMMEDIATELY POSTPARTUM

PROBLEM	TREATMENT
Postpartum bleeding (hemorrhage)___________	___________________________
Other___________________________	___________________________

POSTPARTUM STAY IN HOSPITAL

Number of days in hospital___________________________

MEDICATIONS GIVEN (see chart, pp. 218–220)

REASON	NAME	DATE	DOSAGE	HOW GIVEN
To keep uterus contracted				
To dry up breast milk				
For pain relief				
Iron/vitamins				
For sleep				
To have a bowel movement				
RhoGAM (If Rh negative)				
Other___________				

LAB TESTS TAKEN	DATE	RESULT
Hematocrit		
Other___________		
Other___________		

COMPLICATIONS OR PROBLEMS (specify and describe):

____

____

BLOOD TRANSFUSION: Number of pints given___________

If reaction occurred, describe___________

SIX-WEEK POSTPARTUM PERIOD

| TYPE OF MEDICATION/REASON | NAME | DOSAGE | HOW TO TAKE | | SPECIAL INSTRUC-TIONS |
MEDICATIONS GIVEN TO TAKE AT HOME			HOW OFTEN	WITH/WITH-OUT MEALS	
Iron/Vitamins					
Other_______________					
Other_______________					

CONTRACEPTION TO USE AT HOME (See "Contraceptive History" for more information)
Foam and condoms_______________

Other_______________

RESUMPTION OF SEX
Pain?   Yes_____ No_____

Other problems_______________

POSTPARTUM DANGER SIGNS AND PROBLEMS

NOTIFY YOUR PRACTITIONER!

SYMPTOM	POSSIBLE PROBLEM	DATE
Increased bleeding/clots	May be due to too much activity. If it does not subside with rest, may be a postpartum hemorrhage.	
Pain: Abdominal	May be a uterine infection.	
Vaginal	May be poorly healing episiotomy or hematoma. Some pain is expected but should decrease.	
Perineal	May be poorly healing episiotomy. Some pain is expected but should decrease.	
Rectal	May be hemorrhoids or poorly healing 3rd or 4th degree laceration.	
Leg pain	May be a sign of blood clot in the vein—thrombophlebitis.	
Reddened, swollen, warm, or hardened area on leg *Or* reddened streak along leg, may feel like a rope inside the leg	May be a sign of a blood clot in the vein—thrombophlebitis	
Pain with urination, urinary urgency and frequency	Urinary frequency alone is normal in the postpartum period. Pain on the outside area may be soreness due to episiotomy, lacerations, or abrasions. Internal pain while urinating, along with urgency (a strong feeling that you must urinate) and frequency might be a sign of a urinary-tract infection, especially if you urinate only small amounts.	
Fever/Chills	If mild, may be breast engorgement, but can signify infection after the first 24 hours.	
Foul smelling discharge (lochia)	May be postpartum infection.	

TWO-WEEK POSTPARTUM PRACTITIONER VISIT AFTER A CESAREAN BIRTH

DATE_______________________________

QUESTIONS TO ASK

____

____

____

FINDINGS   COMMENTS

   Incision: Healing?___________   Not healing?_________________________________

   Uterus: Involuting?___________   Not involuting?_______________________________

   Blood pressure:____________

   Other___________________

LABORATORY TESTS   RESULTS

   Hematocrit____________________   ____________________________

   Other________________________   _____________________________

MEDICATIONS GIVEN

MEDICATION	REASON	DOSAGE	SPECIAL INSTRUCTIONS

OTHER TREATMENTS____

DATE OF NEXT VISIT_______________________________________

FOUR- TO SIX-WEEK POSTPARTUM PRACTITIONER VISIT

DATE_______________________________

QUESTIONS TO ASK

____

____

____

FINDINGS

Breasts	Normal_________________	Other______________
Uterus	Involuted?_____________	Not involuted?__________
Perineum	Healing?______________	Not healing?__________
Vagina	Healed?__________ Not healed?________	Muscle tone________
Cesarean incision	Healing?______________	Not healed?____________

Blood pressure___________________________________

Other_______________________________

LABORATORY TESTS   RESULTS

Hematocrit__________   ______________

Pap test (if needed)   ______________

Other__________   ______________

MEDICATIONS GIVEN

MEDICATION	REASON	DOSAGE	SPECIAL INSTRUCTIONS

OTHER TREATMENTS GIVEN___________________________________

CONTRACEPTIVE GIVEN___________________________________
(Also record in section "Contraceptive History," p. 140)

POSTPARTUM DIARY (II)

1st week
2nd week
3rd week
4th week
5th week
6th week

NOTES

5

Childhood

The First Child

THE NEWBORN

All births have an element of uncertainty. Parents wonder whether they will have a girl or boy. They imagine how their baby will look and act. Most of all, they hope their child will be healthy.

This chart is designed to reflect the health of your newborn at birth and soon afterward. All infants should be thoroughly examined within twenty-four hours of delivery.

At one and at five minutes of age, babies are assessed and given an "Apgar score" (named after Dr. Virginia Apgar, the physician who developed the scale). The purpose of this score is to decide what, if any, immediate efforts are needed to help your baby breathe and survive. It also aids in determining how much observation is necessary in the early days of life (the neonatal period).

Apgar scores range from zero to ten. Few babies score ten. There are five categories in which a score of zero to two can be assigned. These are breathing efforts, heart rate, muscle tone, reflex activity, and color (blueness). An Apgar score is not an intelligence score. Neither future health nor future performance in any area can be predicted by Apgar scores alone. Some premature babies, for example, have high Apgars but develop respiratory problems shortly after birth. Other babies have low one-minute Apgars, but are aided in breathing (resuscitated) quickly and have no further problems.

We have asked you to record any resuscitative efforts needed and any abnormal physical findings. Should your baby have a problem, use the accompanying chart, "Problems of the Newborn," to fill in details. Such information will be particularly useful if you change practitioners early in your child's life.

Because feeding is the major task of the newborn, we have included information about responses to early feedings. Difficulty in feeding may be a clue that a medical problem exists. Further investigation is called for.

We've also included laboratory tests taken during the neonatal period and medications and treatments received. All may have a bearing on future health. The medical care of newborns involves many controversial areas. Practitioners often disagree on the need for certain tests and treatments. Parents sometimes disagree with their practitioners. Often parents are confused about what actions are appropriate. For example, some practitioners do extensive, and sometimes dangerous, tests if a baby is suspected of having an infection; antibiotics are sometimes used before an infection is definitely diagnosed. Practitioners who believe in these procedures and treatments feel that diligence in diagnosing and preventing possible infection is worth the risks involved. Others feel that intervention is often hasty and unnecessary and sometimes replaces sound clinical judgment individualized to the infant. It makes sense to discuss your prospective practitioner's or clinic's attitudes toward newborn care and make sure that they are consistent with your own.

Almost every state requires by law that eye medications be given just after birth. This prevents the blindness that occurs in a baby whose mother is infected with gonorrhea. The baby picks up the gonococcus organism during passage through the vagina. Antibiotic drops or ointments are used. A transient side effect may be inflammation of the eye. This is most common with silver nitrate drops. Some parents therefore prefer that ointments be used. However, the National Society for the Prevention of Blindness recommends silver nitrate and some state laws specify the type of medication to be used. In some states, the medication requirement may be waived if parents object to it. Parents often ask that antiobiotic administration be postponed until the baby has bonded with them for at least one hour and will naturally drop off to sleep. Discuss these issues with your practitioner or those in your clinic.

Most practitioners routinely give Vitamin K to newborns. Vitamin K is needed for blood clotting. Its manufacture in the body requires the presence of intestinal bacteria, which newborns do not have. Bleeding problems can occur; they are extremely rare, but can be fatal. Vitamin K is generally given as an injection since it is believed that oral Vitamin K is poorly absorbed. Some parents object to their brand-new baby receiving a shot. Some babies given Vitamin K at the currently routine dosage of one milligram show a greater tendency to develop jaundice than those not given the medication. For these reasons, the administration of Vitamin K is a somewhat controversial issue. If you have strong feelings about it, discuss them with your practitioner to get his or her opinion. Decide together in advance whether your baby should be given Vitamin K.

Certain laboratory tests are also required in many states. These include tests for the metabolic disease phenylketonuria (PKU) and for thyroid disorders. Early detection allows for early treatment, preventing long-term disabilities. Babies should have their blood typed to rule out the possibility of incompatibility with the mother's blood type. If this is present, a baby can develop antibodies to fight his or her own blood.

This problem may range from the mild to the serious. A test called a Coombs test is often done to check for such unusual antibodies in the baby's blood. Other tests, such as one for syphilis, and a blood count may be done. Bilirubin levels may be needed for babies who appear unusually yellow (jaundiced). These tests all require a blood sample, which is drawn from the baby's heel.

This chart can be used to record basic information. If your newborn has a problem, an unusual finding on physical examination or in a laboratory test, use the section "Problems of the Newborn" (p. 258).

IMMEDIATE CONDITION OF THE NEWBORN

DATE OF BIRTH_______________________

TIME OF BIRTH_______________________

APGAR SCORE

   1 minute_______________________

   5 minute_______________________

RESUSCITATION NEEDED (Aids to breathing)

None	_______________	
Stimulation	_______________	
Oxygen	_______________	
Ambu Bag	_______________	(Positive pressure oxygen, similar to mouth-to-mouth)
Other	_______________	(See section "Problems of the Newborn" and specify)

WEIGHT   _______________   (If less than 5½ pounds, see section "Problems of the Newborn—Low Birth Weight")

LENGTH   _______________

CIRCUMFERENCE OF HEAD_______________   CHEST__________   ABDOMEN__________

ESTIMATED GESTATIONAL AGE
(Number of weeks at birth)_______________   (If less than 36 weeks, see "Problems of the Newborn—Prematurity")

Name

NEWBORN PHYSICAL EXAMINATION
To be done within first 24 hours of birth

Name

AREA OF THE BODY	CHECKOFF	
	NORMAL	ABNORMALITY NOTED (SEE SECTION "PROBLEMS OF THE NEWBORN," p. 258)
Head	_________	_________________________
Mouth	_________	_________________________
Nose	_________	_________________________
Eyes	_________	_________________________
Ears	_________	_________________________
Neck	_________	_________________________
Extremities	_________	_________________________
Heart	_________	_________________________
Lungs	_________	_________________________
Abdomen	_________	_________________________
Genitals	_________	_________________________
Spinal Cord	_________	_________________________

BIRTHMARKS: Note location and describe

____

LENGTH OF BABY'S HOSPITAL STAY:

____ Days/Weeks

LABORATORY TESTS TAKEN: If abnormal, see "Problems of the Newborn"

Routine   Blood type   _________________

                 PKU/thyroid   _________________

Other   Hematocrit   _________________

                 Blood glucose   _________________

                 Bilirubin   _________________

                 Other_______________

PROBLEMS (If any, see "Problems of the Newborn")

____

NEWBORN FEEDING

TYPE OF FEEDING
Breast______________________________
Bottle____________________________ Type of formula given_________________

TIME OF FIRST FEEDING________________

RESPONSE TO FIRST FEEDING
Ate well   ____________________
Sleepy   ____________________
Cried   ____________________
Spit up   ____________________
Vomited   ____________________
Other____________ ____________________

RESPONSES TO SUBSEQUENT FEEDINGS
Ate well   ____________________
Sleepy   ____________________
Cried   ____________________
Spit up   ____________________
Vomited   ____________________
Other____________ ____________________

ROOMING-IN   Yes____________   No____________   Partial____________

DEMAND OR SCHEDULE FEEDING:
Demand__________   Schedule________________   Specify schedule__________________

FEEDING PROBLEMS NOTED: _________________________________

(See section "Problems of the Newborn")   _________________________________

Name

PROBLEMS OF THE NEWBORN

Birth is most often a happy event. Sometimes, however, an infant is born with a problem or develops one shortly after birth. Conditions may exist during pregnancy that prepare parents for this, but sometimes it comes as a great shock.

A common and understandable reaction when a child is sick at birth is to ask yourself if you did anything to cause it. Women anguish as they review their every action during and even before their pregnancy, wondering what they could have done differently to have prevented the damage. Fathers and other family members may consciously or unconsciously blame the mother as well. In some families, parents blame each other. Fathers may also feel guilt.

Often, one specific cause cannot be found for a birth defect or illness. Sometimes hereditary factors are significant (see the section "Family History," p. 26). Drugs, chemical exposures, environmental pollutants, and nutritional deficits may play a part, but this cannot always be directly proven. Commonly used substances such as tobacco, caffeine, and alcohol have all been shown to cause problems in newborns, but which babies will be affected cannot always be predicted, although it is known that the more you use, the greater the possibility of damage.

If your newborn has a problem, review your family, medical, obstetrical, and pregnancy histories with your practitioner. The purpose of this is not to find a reason to blame yourself. It is, rather, to help identify possible causes, aid in determining diagnoses, make predictions about the health of future children, and plan preventive measures whenever possible.

At times, large numbers of women in a particular area may deliver babies with similar birth defects. If it can be shown that they have been exposed to the same teratogen (agent causing birth defects), then the cause can be pinpointed. Public pressure can be exerted to change destructive practices of industry or the medical community. Damage suits can be initiated against drug companies, businesses, and even governments.

The emotional upheaval and physical fatigue that ensue following the birth of a sick child can be devastating. Guilt, anger, fear, and sorrow are natural. We urge you to accept all available resources for aid in dealing with emotions. Partners, friends, and relatives can be invaluable. Most likely, you will find that your feelings are shared. Professional help may also be valuable. Feelings may linger for quite a while, especially if your baby dies or is permanently disabled. Such events are not easy to accept.

We encourage parents of premature or ill babies to get as involved as possible in their care. An increasing number of hospitals provide support and teaching to parents who want to participate. Remember, even very tiny and very ill babies benefit from loving attention and physical affection. Before choosing a place for birth, you may want to find out what provisions the hospital (or affiliated hospital in the case of birth centers or home birth) makes for parents to visit and care for sick babies. Make sure these policies are consistent with your values and desires. Use the "Birth Plan for Unexpected Situations" (p. 195) to help you decide what these are. If the region where you live does not allow much choice (has few hospitals or has many but all with similar restrictive practices), we suggest working with other concerned parents to change institutional policies. You often meet parents with similar attitudes in childbirth-education classes.

The charts in this section outline the common areas of problems in newborns. They allow you to detail diagnostic tests, medications, treatments, including surgeries, and any of their exhibited side effects. When deciding how to diagnose or treat a newborn problem, practitioners must weigh risks of procedures against their side effects and against the risks of not treating the suspected or diagnosed condition. We believe parents should be involved in such choices, but these decisions are often difficult to make. An example is whether to treat a rising bilirubin level (see p. 268). The condition must be treated before a dangerous level is reached, yet the currently available treatment—phototherapy (the use of ultraviolet lights)—poses short-term hazards and possible unknown long-term risks (see p. 269). We recommend discussing each of your practitioners' decisions with them, learning the alternatives, and giving your input whenever possible. We acknowledge that when your child is concerned, it can be painful and frightening to be informed. It is not unusual to be afraid to ask questions, to fear the answers. Often, however, knowledge can allay anxiety and help you become part of the team caring for your baby. These charts can provide information that may be significant for your child throughout life. Spend a few moments each day talking to your child's practitioner. Try to find the strength to record necessary information. Use this section to learn more about your baby's condition and progress.

The High-Risk Child: A Guide for Concerned Parents by Philip R. Deppe and Judith L. Sherman with Sydelle Engel (Macmillan Publishing Co., Inc., New York, 1981) is recommended for parents who have a child with a disability. *When Pregnancy Fails* by Susan Borg and Judith Lasker (Beacon Press, Boston, 1981) is a helpful book for parents who experience a miscarriage or a stillbirth or whose child dies in infancy.

PROBLEMS OF THE NEWBORN

Birth weight_________ pounds_________ ounces   Number of weeks gestation_______________
_________________________________grams

SPECIFIC PROBLEM(S) DIAGNOSED PROBLEM	DATE DIAGNOSED	DATE RESOLVED
___________________	___________	___________
___________________	___________	___________
___________________	___________	___________
___________________	___________	___________

DIAGNOSTIC TESTS	DATE	RESULT	DATE	RESULT	DATE	RESULT	SIDE EFFECTS
X rays: Chest							
Other:							
_________							
_________							
Sepsis Work-up (tests for infection) Blood culture							
Culture of nose, ear, throat, any discharge							
Urine culture							
Spinal tap							
Suprapubic (bladder) tap							

DIAGNOSTIC TESTS	DATE	RESULT	DATE	RESULT	DATE	RESULT	SIDE EFFECTS
Blood gases							
pH							
PO_2							
pCO_2							
Complete blood count							
White blood cells							
Red blood cells							
Hemoglobin							
Hematocrit							
Other blood tests							
Bilirubin							
Glucose							
Calcium							
Toxicology (for presence of drugs)							
Other (specify)							
Other tests (specify)							

Name

FEEDING METHODS AND DATES

Tube _____________   Intravenous _____________   _____________

Breast _____________   Bottle _____________   _____________

Other _____________   Name(s) of Formula(s): _____   _____________

_____________   _____________

_____________   _____________

Name ______

MEDICATIONS GIVEN	REASON	DATE(S) BEGAN	ENDED	HOW GIVEN	DOSAGE	NOTED SIDE EFFECTS

TREATMENTS GIVEN	REASON	DATE(S) BEGAN	ENDED	RESULTS	NOTED SIDE EFFECTS
Oxygen (specify if given by respirator and if through mask, nasal prongs, hood, nasopharyngeal tube or endotracheal tube)					
Phototherapy for bilirubin (ultraviolet lights)					
Blood transfusion(s)					
Casts					
Surgeries (describe) ______					
______					
______					
Special exercises (describe) ______					
Other (describe) ______					
______					

QUESTIONS REGARDING IN-HOSPITAL TESTS, MEDICATIONS OR TREATMENTS

Name

NAME AND SPECIALTY OF PRACTITIONER(S) INVOLVED IN CARE

NAME	SPECIALTY

DISCHARGE INFORMATION

Weight when discharged from hospital _______________ pounds _______________ ounces

_______________ grams

Date of discharge_______________

SPECIAL INSTRUCTIONS WHEN BABY GOES HOME_______________

____

____

____

____

____

DATE(S) OF PRACTITIONER VISIT(S):

Pediatrician_______________

Other specialists_______________

____

____

AT HOME

QUESTIONS TO ASK PEDIATRICIAN OR OTHER PRACTITIONERS_______________

____

____

____

____

____

____

____

____

____

Name

NOTES

(Record feelings, baby's responses, behaviors, feeding and sleeping patterns, etc.)

SELECTED PROBLEMS, TESTS, AND TREATMENTS IN THE NEWBORN

PROBLEM	EXPLANATION	COMMON DIAGNOSTIC TESTS
PRE-MATURITY	A baby born earlier than the beginning of the 9th month (36th week) of pregnancy is premature. Can result in serious respiratory problems since baby's lungs are not quite ready to handle the task of breathing. Other problems may arise as well. Premature babies need constant, meticulous supervision.	See: Breathing problems Hyperbilirubinemia Blood chemistry tests: glucose and calcium, for example Complete blood count
LOW BIRTH WEIGHT OR SMALL FOR GESTA-TIONAL AGE (SGA)	A low-birth-weight baby is a baby in the lowest 10th percentile of weight for his or her gestational age (number of weeks at birth). May or may not be premature. May result from intrauterine growth retardation (IUGR) caused by poor maternal nutri-tion, drugs, or disease.	See: Prematurity Breathing problems
BIRTH DE-FECTS AND/OR IN-JURIES (CONGENI-TAL ANOMA-LIES)	Birth defects include cleft lip or palate (harelip), extra or missing fingers or toes or developmental defects of the arms or legs. Defects can occur in any body system or organ, such as heart and circulatory system or digestive or reproductive systems. Some problems, such as deafness, may not be apparent at birth.	X rays Genetic studies (of the baby and parents) Electrocardiogram (EKG)
INFECTION	An infection can occur in any newborn, but is most likely in babies with other problems. Newborn infections may be difficult to diagnose because symptoms are vague and not specific to the area of infection. Infections may easily spread in newborns and enter the bloodstream (sepsis) or cause meningitis—an inflammation of the mem-branes of the brain or spinal cord.	Complete blood count Sepsis work-up Blood culture Culture of nose, ear, throat, or any discharge Urine culture Spinal tap Suprapubic (bladder) tap
BREATHING PROBLEMS	Breathing problems often accompany prematurity. They may, however, occur for other reasons in full-term babies. They include respiratory distress syndrome (RDS), also called hyaline membrane disease (HMD), pneumonia, and meconium aspi-ration (breathing in of the contents of the fetal bowel, before, during, or after birth).	Chest X ray Blood gases pH pO_2 pCO_2
LARGE FOR GESTA-TIONAL AGE (LGA)	Large-for-gestational-age babies may not have problems. These babies, in the upper 10th percen-tile of weight for their gestational age, may simply have a hereditary tendency to largeness. Often, however, they are born to diabetic mothers and do have some problems, particularly low blood-glucose (sugar) levels.	Blood chemistry tests: Glucose Calcium Magnesium

POSSIBLE TEST SIDE EFFECTS	COMMON TREATMENTS	POSSIBLE TREATMENT SIDE EFFECTS
See appropriate sections	Incubation See appropriate sections	
See appropriate sections	May need supplemental feedings See Breathing Problems Treatment depends upon problems that develop	
Long-term effects unknown Any blood test can result in local inflammatory reaction	Varies with problem Casts, corrective exercises, surgeries	Infections Risks of anesthesia if necessary—breathing difficulties
Introduction of infection Spinal tap—pain, trauma, possibly breathing difficulties secondary to trauma Suprapubic tap—damage to the urinary bladder	Antibiotics Isolation	Varies with drug, dosage, length of time given Can cause blood disorders, kidney or ear damage Overgrowth of other infections, such as thrush (yeast) Resistance to the drug
Radiation Infection of umbilical artery—(used to monitor blood gases)	Immediate: Intubation—tube from mouth or nose into trachea (breathing tube) to aid air flow; suction Oxygen, via respirator if unable to breathe on own Heart stimulation—cardiac massage; epinephrine Correction of chemical imbalances—sodium bicarbonate Long-term: may need continuous respiratory support	Overdose of oxygen can cause eye damage Levels must be carefully controlled
	Correction of chemical imbalances May need glucose, calcium, etc., given by mouth or intravenously if necessary	Infection at intravenous site

SELECTED PROBLEMS, TESTS, AND TREATMENTS IN THE NEWBORN (continued)

PROBLEM	EXPLANATION	COMMON DIAGNOSTIC TESTS
JAUNDICE/ HYPER-BILIRUBI-NEMIA	Jaundice is caused by an excess of the chemical bilirubin in the body. Bilirubin is made when red blood cells (RBCs) are destroyed, a normal body process that occurs in adults as well as newborns. Newborns are naturally born with too many RBCs. As the body destroys them, the bilirubin released is usually cleared by the liver. Babies have immature livers and sometimes their livers don't do the job well. This causes jaundice—a yellowing of the skin—as the bilirubin builds up. It becomes a problem when levels get too high. These dangerous levels can result in brain damage called kernicterus. Babies with other problems may be especially likely to develop hyperbilirubinemia.	Bilirubin blood levels
OTHER BLOOD PROBLEMS	Blood disorders in infants include anemia, a reduced number of RBCs, or reduced amount of hemoglobin in the cells. This may be caused by "ABO Incompatibility," a condition that occurs when mother's blood is Type O and baby's is Type A, B, or AB. When this occurs, antibodies that the mother built up against the baby's blood are found in the baby's own bloodstream and attack his or her blood. Another blood problem in newborns is polycythemia—too many RBCs.	Complete blood count
FEEDING PROBLEMS	Feeding problems are usually symptoms of some-thing else—an allergy, a birth defect in the digestive system, a metabolic disorder. They may, however, be "colic," a basically normal though disturbed condition in which a newborn reacts to feeding, often violently, in apparent pain and distress. Time is the only cure for colic, although removing milk or other allergens from a breast-feeding mother's diet may help. All feeding prob-lems require looking into before they can be called colic.	X rays Blood tests for metabolic or allergic problems
INBORN ERRORS OF METABOLISM	There are many disorders involving the body's enzymes—chemical substances used in the diges-tive process. These disorders result in the inability to digest certain substances found in food. Al-though rare, it is important that they can be diagnosed early in life since the elimination of these substances from the diet can prevent further serious problems. The best-known of these is phenylketonuria (PKU) for which all infants are tested early in life.	Blood tests

POSSIBLE TEST SIDE EFFECTS	COMMON TREATMENTS	POSSIBLE TREATMENT SIDE EFFECTS
	Phototherapy—continuous use of ultraviolet lights	Short-term effects include damage to the eyes if not completely covered, dehydration, and loss of maternal contact. Long-term effects not known
	Exchange transfusion	Infection Irregular heartbeats Cardiac (heart) overload Blood clotting Imbalances of body chemicals
	Transfusion may be necessary	Infection
Radiation	Depends on problem diagnosed May need intravenous or tube feeding May need corrective surgery May need special diet	Infection at IV site Risks of anesthesia Risks of poor nutrition
Infection at site of blood test	Dietary changes, such as the elimination of the amino acid phenylalanine in PKU	Emotional difficulties associated with dietary restrictions

INFANT FEEDING

Your decisions on infant feeding will affect both your baby and yourselves. Grandparents on both sides of the family, friends, doctors, nurses, midwives, and other family members can offer you advice (sometimes more than you would wish). Take time to consider your choices.

Breast milk is the ideal infant food, supplying all nutritional needs for the baby's first six months. Certain immunities are passed from the mother to the infant in breast milk. Breast-fed babies have lower rates of intestinal infection and fewer allergies than formula-fed babies do.

Breast-feeding has benefits for the mother also, helping the uterus to return to normal size, encouraging rest, and supplying convenient and constantly available milk. It provides physical enjoyment and closeness for both mother and child.

Breast milk is more easily and quickly digested than formula. Much contradictory advice exists on frequency of breast-feeding, which can be confusing for new parents. Some practitioners and books refer to feedings at four-hour intervals: the 6 A.M., 10 A.M., 2 P.M. feedings, and so on. Most of these references seem to be for the convenience of the author or practitioner, since medical thinking has moved away from rigid scheduling of baby's feedings. Other sources advise nursing every three to four hours, or perhaps every two to three hours. Some will encourage feeding on demand, no matter what the hour. We agree with this.

Many cultural and personal factors will affect your decisions about frequency of nursing. In some cultures, mothers routinely offer the breast whenever the baby cries. Some women who have tried this approach say they found it less work than considering the timing of the feedings, because their babies were easily contented and rarely cried for long. Demand feedings usually average about eight to twelve a day for newborns (equivalent to nursing every two to three hours), although some feedings come much closer together than others. As the baby grows, feedings tend to be spaced farther apart.

It is not uncommon for the mother's nipples to be tender or sore when she first begins to nurse. They will rapidly grow adjusted to the new activity. Avoiding the use of soap or other drying agents on the nipples can help prevent the tenderness.

Most nursing mothers never experience serious problems. Occasionally, however, difficulties do arise. It is best to prevent or to deal immediately with minor difficulties to avoid discomfort. If at any time you experience severe pain, a red spot or streak, a sore lump on the breast, or a fever and feeling of exhaustion, you should contact your practitioner immediately. These may be signs of infection. There is some controversy regarding nursing during breast infections. There is no evidence, however, that shows this to be harmful to mothers or babies. Nursing helps keep the breast empty of milk, which tends to speed recovery.

You have three resources for problem-solving in breast-feeding— your practitioner, your friends and family members who have successfully breast-fed their children, and organizations which support breast-feeding such as the Childbirth Education Association and the La

Leche League. At the end of this chapter, you will find a list of books which provide information on breast-feeding and breast care. If you take medication for any reason, be sure to tell your practitioner you are a nursing mother. You can record all medications and their dates on page 273.

Many parents will wish to give a bottle from time to time, containing either expressed breast milk or formula. Some mothers who return to work while the infant is young give bottles during the day and nurse during evenings, nights, and weekends. The milk supply rapidly adjusts to accommodate a part-time schedule. These parents can use the charts for both breast and formula feedings.

Sometimes mothers do not wish to breast-feed their babies, or after starting the baby on the breast find it difficult or undesirable to continue. There are a wide variety of infant formulas on the market. Formulas can also be prepared at home. Your practitioner will advise you on selecting the proper formula for your baby.

The chart "Formula Feeding Records," page 273, is provided to record brand names of any formula your child takes, with the dates each is given. It is impossible to duplicate mother's milk exactly, and sometimes formula components are changed. There have been instances of recall of infant formulas, and you may need to know in the future exactly at what time your child was on a particular formula.

The question of whether or not to give supplementary vitamins to breast-fed babies is another controversial one. Some practitioners believe that breast-fed babies should be given vitamins A, C, and D, plus fluoride and iron, since these are lacking or present at low levels in breast milk. Others point to the fact that vitamin deficiency is rare in breast-fed babies as long as the mother eats a balanced diet, and they do not recommend supplements except under special circumstances. Formula-fed babies do not need supplements, although they should be fed iron-fortified formula after the first few months.

Infants do not need solid food added to their diets until they are six months old, though advertisements for baby cereals and some literature refer to feeding at two to four months. This is another sensitive area. Some relatives may feel you are starving your baby by waiting until six months to introduce solids. Twenty to thirty years ago, children were often fed pureed foods at the age of two weeks—even, occasionally, from birth. Now, medical opinion has turned toward later feeding. It seems to create fewer allergies. The baby's digestive system is more mature and ready to handle different foods. Another advantage for the parents is that it is considerably easier to start solids later. There is no need for expensive baby foods. Few foods even need to be pureed; instead, mashing with a fork is usually sufficient. The baby can soon begin eating "finger foods," which are easily picked up and easy to chew.

Solid foods should be introduced gradually, one at a time, about a week apart. The one-week intervals allow you to detect the problem food if an allergic reaction develops. For more information, see "Allergy," page 278.

Do not be concerned if the baby is not an enthusiastic eater at first. You should not feel competitive with the mothers of other babies or make comparisons between your children. Babies are little individuals, and some take longer to develop an interest in solid foods than others do. By eighteen months, the baby will probably be eating three meals a day and a balanced diet. Some children, however, balance their diets not as adults do—by eating several foods at one meal—but by eating a variety of foods, one or two each meal, within a few days. This is perfectly acceptable. Consult your practitioner if you are concerned about your child's nutrition.

We have not included any charts for introducing solid foods. It is easy to write on a calendar, a week apart, the foods you plan on introducing. This way you can be sure a variety of foods are included, and you can easily check back in case of allergy.

Several basic baby books give general nutrition information. For further information on breast feeding, see *The Complete Book of Breast Feeding* by Marvin Eiger, M.D., and Sally Olds (Bantam Books, New York, 1973). Also see *The Womanly Art of Breastfeeding* from La Leche League International (Franklin Park, Illinois, 1982) and *Nursing Your Baby* by Karen Pryor (Harper & Row, New York, 1963). A medical text that is not too difficult for the average reader is *Breastfeeding—A Guide for the Medical Profession* by Ruth Lawrence (C. V. Mosby, St. Louis, 1980).

BREAST-FEEDING RECORDS

Medications Taken by Breast-Feeding Mother					
NAME OF MEDICATION	**DOSAGE & HOW OFTEN**	**REASON**	**DOCTOR (IF BY PRESCRIPTION)**	**DATES TAKEN**	**REACTIONS IN MOTHER OR BABY**

Difficulties and Relief Measures Taken		
DISCOMFORT OR DIFFICULTY (e.g., sore nipples)	**RELIEF MEASURES—NOTES**	**DATES**

FORMULA-FEEDING RECORDS

Brand of formula____

Date introduced_______________________ Date stopped______________

Reactions____

Brand of formula____

Date introduced_______________________ Date stopped______________

Reactions____

Brand of formula____

Date introduced_______________________ Date stopped______________

Reactions____

Date introduced to cow's milk__________________________________

Reactions____

NOTES

CHILD DEVELOPMENT

Every baby is a unique individual. We have deliberately *not* included any "standards of normal development" charts. The rates of development among perfectly healthy babies span a wide range and are influenced by many factors. We think of all babies as being the same age at birth, but in fact maturity may vary by weeks from the date of conception. "Average" development charts sometimes leave parents with anxiety about a child who seems to be "behind schedule." The statistically average baby is just that—a statistic, not a living creature.

You can, however, record some of your baby's developmental milestones and important "first" events in the pages that follow. We have also included a chart of behaviors that sometimes cause anxiety for parents but in fact are common in normal, healthy children. It can be reassuring to know that all children experience certain difficult stages in life, such as the rebelliousness of the two-year-old. Finally, we have included a list of symptoms that can indicate possible difficulties in the early months. If you have serious questions or fears about your child's development, consult your practitioner.

There have been numerous books written about child development. Most include attitudes on parenting that reflect the views and culture of their authors. They are useful, however, for practical advice when you need it. Ultimately, you must make your own judgments. There is, of course, the classic *Baby and Child Care* by Benjamin Spock, M.D. (Pocket Books, New York, 1976).

Other good references are *Child's Body: A Parent's Manual* by the Diagram Group (Bantam Books, New York, 1979); *The Parenting Advisor* by Frank Caplan, Princeton Center for Infancy (Anchor Books, New York, 1978); and *Infants and Mothers* by T. Berry Brazelton, M.D. (Delacorte Press, New York, 1972).

ACHIEVEMENTS AND MILESTONES

FIRST TIME CHILD . . .	DATE	AGE	NOTES AND COMMENTS
Smiled			
Lifted head			
Turned over—front to back			
back to front			
Held head erect			
Laughed			
First tooth			
Sat up			
Crawled			
Stood up			
First kiss			
Walked with help			
Walked alone			
Drank from cup			
Used spoon			
First words			
Said family names			
First phrases			
Recognized shapes			
Recognized letters			

Name

NORMAL BEHAVIORS THAT CAN CREATE WORRY FOR PARENTS

BEHAVIOR	AGES	COMMENTS
Waking at night	9 months to 1 year; periodically through second year	Usually caused by teething. Pinworms and ear problems are also possible causes.
Separation anxiety (fear when the parent leaves the child's sight)	Begins at 11 to 14 months; usually ends at about 18 months	Develops at about the same time as walking and may help keep toddlers from getting lost.
Masturbation (playing with genitals)	1 year 3 years throughout childhood	Self-exploration, curiosity, pleasure: it feels good. Occasionally caused by need to urinate or presence of rash or genital irritation.
Rebelliousness, running away when called, etc.	18 months to 2 years	An effort by the child to declare his independence and strike out alone.
Dawdling	2 to 2½ years	Caused by child's different interests and also by rebelliousness. Allow more time, or be prepared to carry the dawdler along.
"Late" toilet training	There is no normal age for toilet training.	Does not mean child is bad, stupid, or suffering a physical problem. After the age of three, may be symptom of some difficulty.
Nightmares	Beginning at about 3 to 5 years	Children today encounter many frightening influences, especially television, which can lead to nightmares. Bad dreams also arise from the stress of life's ordinary anxieties.
Bed-wetting	Up to about age 4 to 5 years	Some children are not dry at night until 5. After this age, may be allergy, sleep disorders, or other causes.

SIGNALS OF POSSIBLE DEVELOPMENTAL PROBLEMS

In the early months, these symptoms can be caused by a range of problems including colic or even simple gas pains, allergy, brain damage, inadequate milk intake, and many other factors. If one or another of these descriptions persistently applies to your child, it calls for a visit to the child's practitioner. Only a trained practitioner can distinguish between the many possible causes and make sure correct treatment is begun.

Babies who seem to have no need of their mother (sometimes described as being "too good")

Babies who seem as if they would rather not be touched (crying or struggling when they are picked up)

Babies who cry *constantly* and cannot be consoled

Babies who arch the back and scream when they are touched

Babies who do not begin to make contact with the parents, who avoid meeting the parents' eyes

Babies who fail to gain weight or grow (failure to thrive)

ALLERGY

If you have listened to parents of young children comparing notes, allergy was probably a frequent topic. It is a common and serious medical problem, with reactions ranging from low-level irritation to life-threatening danger. There are strong hereditary tendencies toward developing allergies. Environmental factors, stress, and the exposure of the fetus to various foods and drugs are also contributing factors. You should consult your practitioner if you suspect allergy in your child.

Allergy is an overreaction by the body to a given substance (the "allergen"). Normally, a food is digested and its components broken down either to be used by the body's cells or to be eliminated. When a food or other substance cannot be tolerated within the body, the presence of its by-products triggers the production of antibodies, as if infection were present. During this process, a chemical called "histamine" is released in the cells. The symptoms of allergy show themselves wherever histamine is present. If it is released in the skin, a rash appears; if in the digestive system, diarrhea or other gastric symptoms may result.

No one can have an allergic reaction the first time he or she is exposed to a substance. Only after the initial exposure does antibody formation and sensitization take place. Reactions usually show within the next several exposures, though it is possible to develop an allergy to a substance that was previously tolerated. Allergies may disappear after a number of years, or they may remain lifelong.

Common allergic reactions in children include eczema, rashes, diarrhea, hives, and many other symptoms. Some allergies may have an effect on behavior or learning. Children who are thought to be overactive (hyperkinetic) or learning-disabled may be behaving badly because of allergy. Bad temper or a lack of energy might even be caused by allergy. You can imagine the situation of a child who is allergic to wheat but has always eaten bread—thinking that stomachaches or consistent headaches are a normal condition of life.

Allergies to a vast number of substances have been recorded. Some of the most common and best known include allergies to environmental substances such as pollen, grass, or house dust, food allergies, and allergies to insect stings. Measures for treatment and relief include eliminating the allergen, desensitization treatments, nutrition plans, and measures to reduce stress. It may be necessary to consult a specialist in the treatment of allergies.

Sometimes a child is diagnosed as having a milk intolerance (lactose intolerance). This is not the same as an allergy. Lactose is the form of sugar which naturally occurs in milk. Some children (and many adults) do not produce the enzyme which is used to digest lactose. Lactose is present in many foods, and special dietary planning is usually necessary for people who cannot digest it.

To help detect food allergies in young children, new foods should be started in the diet one at a time, about a week apart. If a reaction develops, it will usually be to the food that has been introduced most recently. It is possible, however, for allergy to develop later on.

Two of the charts that follow are worksheets to help discover the food causing a reaction. On the first, you can check off the appearance of symptoms with the appearance of foods in the diet. This worksheet lists common allergies and leaves room for you to include those suspected by yourself and your practitioner. On the second worksheet, you can keep track of the dates a possible allergen is removed from the diet, whether the symptoms cleared, and reactions when the food was eaten again.

This section also provides a chart to record all diagnosed allergies, dates and nature of reactions, treatment, and results. This is important information which should be available to any practitioner your child sees.

ALLERGY DETECTION WORKSHEET (I)

Name

POSSIBLE ALLERGEN	SUN	MON	TUE	WED	THU	FRI	SAT	SUN	MON	TUE	WED	THU	FRI	SAT
Milk—and yogurt, cheese, butter														
Egg (especially egg white)														
Corn														
Wheat—and bread, noodles, cereal														
Chocolate														
Pork (including bacon, ham, sausage)														
Tomatoes and juice														
Oranges and juice														
Spinach														
Peanut butter														
SYMPTOMS														
Hives														
Diarrhea														
Eczema														
Rash														

ALLERGY DETECTION WORKSHEET (I)

POSSIBLE ALLERGEN	REACTION	DATE ELIMINATED FROM DIET	DATE SYMPTOMS CLEARED	DATE INTRODUCED AGAIN	RESULTS AND NOTES

Name _______________

RECORD OF ALLERGIES

Name _______________

ALLERGEN	REACTION(S)	DATE(S) REACTION NOTED	TREATMENT/ RELIEF MEASURES	DATES	RESULTS

IMMUNIZATION

Immunization is one of the most extensive public-health programs carried out across the United States. In almost every community, free immunizations have been available to children regardless of income level or whether the child usually attends a clinic or sees a private practitioner. The development of the immunization program has been one factor in the lowering of the infant and child mortality rate during this century.

The vaccines routinely given to infants and children protect against the following diseases: polio, diphtheria, tetanus, pertussis (whooping cough), measles, mumps, and rubella (German measles). Most are given by injection. Polio vaccine, however, is given by mouth. It is called "trivalent oral polio vaccine." The word "trivalent" means it is effective against three different strains of polio virus.

Recently some practitioners and health consumers who are one segment of the noninterventionist trend in health care have begun to write and speak against routine immunization of children. They argue that with polio, for example, as many cases are traceable to side effects of immunization as occur among nonimmunized children. They say that certain religious groups whose beliefs forbid immunization have not experienced polio epidemics.

We consider these arguments dangerous and strongly suggest you make sure your children are immunized. The lack of disease among nonimmunized children is not a good argument when they live in a larger society surrounded by children who have been immunized, thus making exposure to the disease unlikely.

Disease can be defeated through widespead public immunization programs; recently, smallpox was declared to be extinct, thanks to immunization. But until this process has been completed on a broad, even international, scale, the threat of infection remains. Immunization against these serious diseases of childhood protects your child and helps prevent future epidemics.

The Record of Immunizations shows the age at which each is usually given. The schedule of your practitioner or clinic should resemble this list closely but may vary slightly.

RECORD OF IMMUNIZATIONS

Name

VACCINE	DOSE	DATE	PRACTITIONER OR CLINIC	REACTION
Diphtheria-Pertussis (Whooping Cough)- Tetanus (DPT)	1st (2 mo.)			
	2nd (4 mo.)			
	3rd (6 mo.)			
	4th (18 mo.)			
	5th (4 to 5 yrs.)			
Trivalent Oral Polio Vaccine	1st (2 mo.)			
	2nd (4 mo.)			
	3rd (6 mo.)			
	4th (4 to 5 yrs.)			
Measles-Mumps-Rubella (German Measles) (MMR)	15 mo.			
Tetanus-Diphtheria	1st (14 to 15 mo.)			
	booster			
	booster			
	booster			
Other				

CHILDHOOD PRACTITIONER VISITS

Several factors can be part of your selection of a practitioner to care for your child. You may decide to select a pediatrician in private practice or to have your baby cared for through a well-baby clinic. You may take the child to the family doctor, who might be a general practitioner or a specialist in family practice. Some clinics combine family practice with other specialties or with the services of physicians' assistants and nurse-practitioners. Often, there is more than one clinic that your child would be eligible to attend.

If you have an opportunity to discuss matters with your practitioner or practitioners in advance, there are a few questions it is wise to cover. You will probably wish to find someone who is close to you in philosophy. Ask their opinion on methods of infant feeding, and compare it to your own. Find out, through direct discussion or through friends and other patients, whether they tend to be aggressive in treatment or whether they are noninterventionist in philosophy. It is also a good idea to ask with which hospital they are affiliated and to discuss money—including regular fees, and fees for special services such as attending a Cesarean section. How accessible they are during non-office hours is important to know as well.

Your child's practitioner will be contributing advice and care to your family for years to come. He or she will also be able to refer you to other specialists, should they be needed. Take the time to find a practitioner you trust and will work well with.

PRACTITIONER VISITS AND HOSPITALIZATIONS

DATE	PRACTITIONER, CLINIC OR HOSPITAL/ NAME AND ADDRESS	WEIGHT AND LENGTH/ HEIGHT	REASON FOR VISIT	DIAGNOSTIC TESTS AND RESULTS*	PRACTITIONER'S DIAGNOSIS

Name

* Include yearly TB skin tests.

QUESTIONS FOR PRACTITIONER	TREATMENT OR MEDICATION			INSTRUCTIONS	REACTIONS OR COMMENTS
	NAME	HOW OFTEN?	WITH MEALS?		

Name

PRACTITIONER VISITS AND HOSPITALIZATIONS

Name ___________

DATE	PRACTITIONER, CLINIC OR HOSPITAL/ NAME AND ADDRESS	WEIGHT AND LENGTH/ HEIGHT	REASON FOR VISIT	DIAGNOSTIC TESTS AND RESULTS*	PRACTITIONER'S DIAGNOSIS

* Include yearly TB skin tests.

QUESTIONS FOR PRACTITIONER	TREATMENT OR MEDICATION			INSTRUCTIONS	REACTIONS OR COMMENTS
	NAME	HOW OFTEN?	WITH MEALS?		

Name ________________

DENTAL VISITS

Name

DATE	NAME AND ADDRESS OF PRACTITIONER	REASON FOR VISIT (E.G., CHECKUP, TOOTHACHE, BLEEDING GUMS, ETC.)	QUESTIONS TO ASK	NO. OF X RAYS	ABDOMINAL SHIELD USED?

TREATMENTS/ MEDICATIONS/ ANESTHESIA (E.G., FILLINGS, EXTRACTIONS, NITROUS OXIDE, ETC.)	POST-TREATMENT MEDICATIONS			REACTIONS NOTED	SPECIAL REFERRALS/ INSTRUCTIONS
	NAME	HOW OFTEN	SPECIAL INSTRUCTIONS		

Name

EYE-CARE VISITS

Name

Date and Location of First Vision Testing _______________

DATE	PRACTITIONER NAME AND ADDRESS	REASON FOR VISIT	QUESTIONS TO ASK

Vision at first testing ____

RESULTS OF EYE EXAM	TREATMENTS (EYEGLASSES, EXERCISES, ETC.)	REFERRALS	SPECIAL INSTRUCTIONS

Name

RECORD OF X RAYS

Name

DATE	REASON	AREA(S) X-RAYED & NUMBER OF EXPOSURES & RADS (ASK RADIOLOGIST OR TECHNICIAN)	RESULT/ DIAGNOSIS	NAME & ADDRESS OF PRACTITIONER AND/OR HOSPITAL

OTHER DIAGNOSTIC TESTS
(See p. 91 for section of common diagnostic tests)

TEST	DATE	REASON	PRACTITIONER	HOSPITAL/ CLINIC/OFFICE	RESULT

Name

SOME COMMONLY USED MEDICATIONS IN CHILDHOOD
(excluding vaccines)

TYPE OF DRUG	CHEMICAL (GENERIC) NAME	EXAMPLES OF BRAND NAMES	HOW GIVEN/ DOSAGE
TO FIGHT BACTE-RIAL INFECTIONS: ANTIBIOTICS	Many, many antibiotics Examples: Penicillin, ampicillin, other "cillin" drugs Erythromycin and other "mycin" drugs Tetracycline	Omnipen Amoxil Erythrocin Kantrex Cleocin	By mouth, IM, IV, for serious infections requiring hospitalization. Dosage varies with illness and medication. Usually given every 6 hours for 10 to 14 days.
NUTRITIONAL SUPPLEMENTS: MULTIVITAMINS FLUORIDES IRON	Vitamins A, D, C Vitamins A, D, C with fluoride Multivitamins with fluoride with iron	Tri-Vi-Sol Tri-Vi-Flor Poly-Vi-Sol Poly-Vi-Flor Poly-Vi-Sol with iron	By mouth, drops, 1 ml every day to age 3; then chewables, one tablet every day.
TO RELIEVE PAIN AND REDUCE FEVER	Acetylsalicylic acid (ASA) Acetaminophen	Many brands of aspirin Tylenol	Varies with age; use pediatric aspirin; check with pharmacist or practitioner. Same as above.

POSSIBLE SIDE EFFECTS	COMMENTS

Short-term:
  Diarrhea, skin rashes, nausea and vomiting
Long-term:
  Ear damage, kidney damage, blood disorders
Development of secondary infection
Development of resistance to medication
Sensitivity to medication
	Do not give to child with a previous sensitivity. Ineffective against viral infections.
	
	Tetracycline should not be used in young children (or during pregnancy) because it will stain the teeth and bones.

With iron—possible constipation	Formula-fed babies need supplementation with A, D, and C. Breast-fed babies need Vitamin C. Both need fluoride only in those states where water is not fortified with fluoride. Fluoride prevents tooth decay. Formula-fed babies need iron only if not given in formula. Do not give two sources of iron.
Stomach upsets Internal bleeding Overdose can cause respiratory depression.	Take with meals. Do not give aspirin to children with diagnosed or suspected chicken pox or after such exposure or during the outbreaks.

ADOLESCENCE

There are no separate charts in this book for the adolescent years. This is not an oversight, nor does it mean that we don't value record-keeping during this life stage. The childhood practitioner-visit charts can be maintained throughout adolescence. We believe that other records reflecting the special needs of the teenage years should be kept by teenagers themselves, in a separate book or on separate pages, for their personal use.

The adolescent years can be a time to learn about taking responsibility for one's own health. As a teenager's body grows and develops into maturity, concern for its well-being can be instilled, partially through instructions about the value of record-keeping. Adolescent girls, for example, should be taught to keep menstrual histories and do breast self-examinations. Both boys and girls need information about contraception; teenage pregnancy is a too-frequent reality in our society. All sections in this book have been written so that they can be understood by most high-school students, who can be shown how to keep their own records. Since teenagers are often quite self-conscious, privacy of records must be assured.

Nutrition is an often-ignored subject among adolescents. The media typically depict teenagers drinking soda, eating at fast-food restaurants, or snacking on empty-calorie foods. Fortunately, healthy eating has recently developed its own popular image. Using the nutritional charts, teenagers can learn to increase awareness of their eating habits. Our culture's emphasis on trim, healthy-looking bodies can be used to motivate good eating habits, although a balance must be maintained so that fad diets will be avoided. We realize that this may be quite a challenge! Exercise is an area in which adolescents often have great interest. They may be eager to keep these records.

Adolescents are usually inquisitive, wanting to know everything. They want, and need, to test their budding independence. This is a good time for them to develop their own relationships with health practitioners. Indeed, in many states, parental consent is not required to provide services for adolescents for venereal disease, birth control, and abortion. The desire to keep records of their health-care visits can foster effective communication with care-givers. Often, school admission requires physical examinations and tests such as chest X rays. Sometimes, needless repetition of such tests can be avoided by having accurate records. This can be especially valuable if schools are changed frequently.

Adolescents eventually grow up and establish their own homes. Before your children leave you, spend some time reviewing with them each parent's family history. Their own birth and childhood histories should be discussed. Perhaps even pregnancy, birth, and postpartum diaries can be shared. The appropriate records can be copied and given to them.

The adolescent years are often turbulent—for parents as well—and always challenging. With proper guidance, positive lifelong health habits can be developed. Record-keeping can become one of these.

Ourselves and Our Children by the Boston Women's Health Collective (Random House, New York, 1978) has a chapter on being the parent of an adolescent. It also lists many other references and resources for parents.

Changing Bodies, Changing Lives is "A Book for Teens on Sex and Relationships" by Ruth Bell and other coauthors of *Our Bodies, Ourselves* and *Ourselves and Our Children* together with members of the Teen-book Project, Random House, 1980. It is recommended for adolescents.

The Second Child

THE SECOND NEWBORN

Although labor, delivery, and birth are now familiar to you, your second newborn is as unique as your first—a totally new creation. She or he looks different, has special characteristics and behaviors. Different problems may arise as well.

It may be especially difficult to accept medical problems in a second child when the first was perfectly healthy. Also, available time and baby-sitters for you to visit a hospitalized newborn may be hard to arrange. You may feel torn apart, trying to give enough to both your children.

Again, we stress that most often the arrival of a newborn is a joyous occasion. The chart "Problems of the Newborn" will remain blank in most books the first time and the second time. For this reason, we have not repeated it. If your second child has a problem, use the chart provided in the first newborn section (pages 260 to 263).

IMMEDIATE CONDITION OF THE NEWBORN (II)

DATE OF BIRTH________________________

TIME OF BIRTH________________________

APGAR SCORE

  1 minute________________________

  5 minute________________________

RESUSCITATION NEEDED (Aids to breathing)

None ________________________

Stimulation ________________________

Oxygen ________________________

Ambu Bag ________________________ (Positive pressure oxygen, similar to mouth-to-mouth)

Other ________________________ (See section "Problems of the Newborn" and specify)

WEIGHT ________________________ (If less than 5½ pounds, see section "Problems of the Newborn—Low Birth Weight")

LENGTH ________________________

CIRCUMFERENCE OF HEAD________________ CHEST__________ ABDOMEN__________

ESTIMATED GESTATIONAL AGE
(Number of weeks at birth)________________ (If less than 36 weeks, see "Problems of the Newborn—Prematurity")

Name

NEWBORN PHYSICAL EXAMINATION (II)
To be done within first 24 hours of birth

Name

AREA OF THE BODY	CHECKOFF	
	NORMAL	ABNORMALITY NOTED (SEE SECTION "PROBLEMS OF THE NEWBORN," p. 258)
Head		
Mouth		
Nose		
Eyes		
Ears		
Neck		
Extremities		
Heart		
Lungs		
Abdomen		
Genitals		
Spinal Cord		

BIRTHMARKS: Note location and describe

____

LENGTH OF BABY'S HOSPITAL STAY:

____ Days/Weeks

LABORATORY TESTS TAKEN: If abnormal, see "Problems of the Newborn"

Routine   Blood type   _______________

                  PKU/thyroid   _______________

Other   Hematocrit   _______________

                  Blood glucose   _______________

                  Bilirubin   _______________

                  Other_____________ _______________

PROBLEMS (If any, see "Problems of the Newborn")

____

NEWBORN FEEDING (II)

TYPE OF FEEDING
  Breast____
  Bottle_____________________________________ Type of formula given__________________

TIME OF FIRST FEEDING________________

RESPONSE TO FIRST FEEDING
  Ate well   ____________________
  Sleepy   ____________________
  Cried   ____________________
  Spit up   ____________________
  Vomited   ____________________
  Other____________ ____________________

RESPONSES TO SUBSEQUENT FEEDINGS
  Ate well   ____________________
  Sleepy   ____________________
  Cried   ____________________
  Spit up   ____________________
  Vomited   ____________________
  Other____________ ____________________

ROOMING-IN   Yes____________   No____________   Partial____________

DEMAND OR SCHEDULE FEEDING:
  Demand__________   Schedule____________   Specify schedule__________________

FEEDING PROBLEMS NOTED: ________________________________

(See section "Problems of the Newborn")   ________________________________

Name

BREAST-FEEDING RECORDS (II)

Medications Taken by Breast-Feeding Mother

NAME OF MEDICATION	DOSAGE & HOW OFTEN	REASON	DOCTOR (IF BY PRESCRIPTION)	DATES TAKEN	REACTIONS IN MOTHER OR BABY

Difficulties and Relief Measures Taken

DISCOMFORT OR DIFFICULTY (e.g., sore nipples)	RELIEF MEASURES—NOTES	DATES

FORMULA-FEEDING RECORDS (II)

Brand of formula____

Date introduced_______________________ Date stopped_______________

Reactions____

Brand of formula____

Date introduced_______________________ Date stopped_______________

Reactions____

Brand of formula____

Date introduced_______________________ Date stopped_______________

Reactions____

Date introduced to cow's milk______________________________________

Reactions____

NOTES

Name

ACHIEVEMENTS AND MILESTONES (II)

FIRST TIME CHILD . . .	DATE	AGE	NOTES AND COMMENTS
Smiled			
Lifted head			
Turned over—front to back			
back to front			
Held head erect			
Laughed			
First tooth			
Sat up			
Crawled			
Stood up			
First kiss			
Walked with help			
Walked alone			
Drank from cup			
Used spoon			
First words			
Said family names			
First phrases			
Recognized shapes			
Recognized letters			

Name

ALLERGY DETECTION WORKSHEET (II)

Name ___________

POSSIBLE ALLERGEN	SUN	MON	TUE	WED	THU	FRI	SAT	SUN	MON	TUE	WED	THU	FRI	SAT
Milk—and yogurt, cheese, butter														
Egg (especially egg white)														
Corn														
Wheat—and bread, noodles, cereal														
Chocolate														
Pork (including bacon, ham, sausage)														
Tomatoes and juice														
Oranges and juice														
Spinach														
Peanut butter														

SYMPTOMS	SUN	MON	TUE	WED	THU	FRI	SAT	SUN	MON	TUE	WED	THU	FRI	SAT
Hives														
Diarrhea														
Eczema														
Rash														

ALLERGY DETECTION WORKSHEET (II)

POSSIBLE ALLERGEN	REACTION	DATE ELIMINATED FROM DIET	DATE SYMPTOMS CLEARED	DATE INTRODUCED AGAIN	RESULTS AND NOTES

Name

RECORD OF ALLERGIES (II)

Name

ALLERGEN	REACTION(S)	DATE(S) REACTION NOTED	TREATMENT/ RELIEF MEASURES	DATES	RESULTS

RECORD OF IMMUNIZATIONS (II)

VACCINE	DOSE	DATE	PRACTITIONER OR CLINIC	REACTION
Diphtheria-Pertussis (Whooping Cough)-Tetanus (DPT)	1st (2 mo.)			
	2nd (4 mo.)			
	3rd (6 mo.)			
	4th (18 mo.)			
	5th (4 to 5 yrs.)			
Trivalent Oral Polio Vaccine	1st (2 mo.)			
	2nd (4 mo.)			
	3rd (6 mo.)			
	4th (4 to 5 yrs.)			
Measles-Mumps-Rubella (German Measles) (MMR)	15 mo.			
Tetanus-Diphtheria	1st (14 to 15 mo.)			
	booster			
	booster			
	booster			
Other				

Name ________________

PRACTITIONER VISITS AND HOSPITALIZATIONS (II)

Name

DATE	PRACTITIONER, CLINIC OR HOSPITAL/ NAME AND ADDRESS	WEIGHT AND LENGTH/ HEIGHT	REASON FOR VISIT	DIAGNOSTIC TESTS AND RESULTS*	PRACTITIONER'S DIAGNOSIS

* Include yearly TB skin tests.

| QUESTIONS FOR PRACTITIONER | TREATMENT OR MEDICATION | | | INSTRUCTIONS | REACTIONS OR COMMENTS |
	NAME	HOW OFTEN?	WITH MEALS?		

Name ___________

PRACTITIONER VISITS AND HOSPITALIZATIONS (II)

Name ____________

DATE	PRACTITIONER, CLINIC OR HOSPITAL/ NAME AND ADDRESS	WEIGHT AND LENGTH/ HEIGHT	REASON FOR VISIT	DIAGNOSTIC TESTS AND RESULTS*	PRACTITIONER'S DIAGNOSIS

* Include yearly TB skin tests.

QUESTIONS FOR PRACTITIONER	TREATMENT OR MEDICATION			INSTRUCTIONS	REACTIONS OR COMMENTS
	NAME	HOW OFTEN?	WITH MEALS?		

Name

DENTAL VISITS (II)

Name

DATE	NAME AND ADDRESS OF PRACTITIONER	REASON FOR VISIT (E.G., CHECKUP, TOOTHACHE, BLEEDING GUMS, ETC.)	QUESTIONS TO ASK	NO. OF X RAYS	ABDOMINAL SHIELD USED?

| TREATMENTS/ MEDICATIONS/ ANESTHESIA (E.G., FILLINGS, EXTRACTIONS, NITROUS OXIDE, ETC.) | POST-TREATMENT MEDICATIONS | | | REACTIONS NOTED | SPECIAL REFERRALS/ INSTRUCTIONS |
	NAME	HOW OFTEN	SPECIAL INSTRUC-TIONS		

Name

EYE-CARE VISITS (II)

Date and Location of First Vision Testing _______________________________

DATE	PRACTITIONER NAME AND ADDRESS	REASON FOR VISIT	QUESTIONS TO ASK

Name

Vision at first testing _______________________

RESULTS OF EYE EXAM	TREATMENTS (EYEGLASSES, EXERCISES, ETC.)	REFERRALS	SPECIAL INSTRUCTIONS

Name ___________

RECORD OF X RAYS (II)

DATE	REASON	AREA(S) X-RAYED & NUMBER OF EXPOSURES & RADS *(ASK RADIOLOGIST OR TECHNICIAN)*	RESULT/ DIAGNOSIS	NAME & ADDRESS OF PRACTITIONER AND/OR HOSPITAL

Name _______________

OTHER DIAGNOSTIC TESTS (II)
(See p. 91 for section of common diagnostic tests)

TEST	DATE	REASON	PRACTITIONER	HOSPITAL/ CLINIC/OFFICE	RESULT

Name

EMERGENCY PHONE NUMBERS